GETTIN

GETTING PHYSICAL

A Teenage Health Guide

Dr Aric Sigman

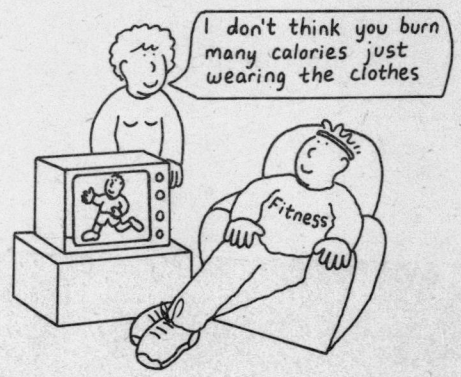

BBC BOOKS

Published by BBC Books,
a division of BBC Enterprises Limited,
Woodlands, 80 Wood Lane
London W12 0TT

First Published 1992
© Aric Sigman 1992

ISBN 0 563 36767 9

Illustrations © Kate Taylor

Typeset by Phoenix Photosetting, Chatham, Kent
Printed and bound in Great Britain by Clays Ltd, St Ives plc
Cover printed by Clays Ltd, St Ives plc

Contents

	Introduction	7
1	Spots	9
2	Suntanning	23
3	Weight and Body Shape	36
4	Food	48
5	Fear of Food	63
6	Unhappiness	76
7	The Way It Is	86
8	Improving Exam Performance	100
9	Getting Physical	110
	Index	123

Introduction

Most people want to know more about health, not because they're interested in trying to prevent the fatal consequences of heart disease, but because they want to feel good, and be happy, confident human beings. Unfortunately, most of their 'information' does not come from objective sources but from those who have something to sell. Somehow science and good professional advice have got lost in the stampede for style, fashion and marketing–hype, designed to gain your attention, trust and money.

Getting Physical is not the typical, comfortable, 'you know it makes sense' health book that many people in the UK have come to expect. It is really an extension of what I do on *Going Live!* – replacing myths with fact, enabling you to make your own choices and to help yourselves. You can rest assured that neither I, nor *Going Live!*, have been sponsored by any organisations to say positive things about their products, services or ideas. Being independent, I am able to present the facts without bias.

Chapter 3, 'Weight and Body Shape' and Chapter 4, 'Food', are a good example of this. The entire issue of weight has been dominated and contaminated by the diet industry, women's magazines and food manufacturers and is often discussed by 'celebrities' who don't know the difference between a carbohydrate and a cosmetic. Having a healthy weight and body shape is remarkably simple and shouldn't cost you a penny, or make you hungry.

Spots are another health topic which is terribly misunderstood. Advertisements falsely depict 'germs' and 'dirt' invading and clogging the pores. Such myths lead you to waste hundreds of millions of pounds on well-known products, most of which do not work. However, chapter one will provide you with a full range of treatments which *do* work.

Our society still tends to be reluctant to discuss sex openly and honestly so that health messages can get distorted and confused. Information about sex also seems to say 'if you really *must* do it, watch out because you could die later and for heaven's sake, please try not to enjoy it more than is absolutely necessary'! You will find the section on sex presents the facts without judgement.

Finally, I'd like to mention that although 'health' is a somewhat dull and general term, this book contains something interesting and useful for everyone. If you only choose to read one chapter in this book then I would urge you to make it the last chapter on exercise. There are more benefits to be had from exercise than from anything else – and there are more ways to get your exercise than you may have realised.

So *Get Physical*!

Dr Aric Sigman

Chapter 1
Spots

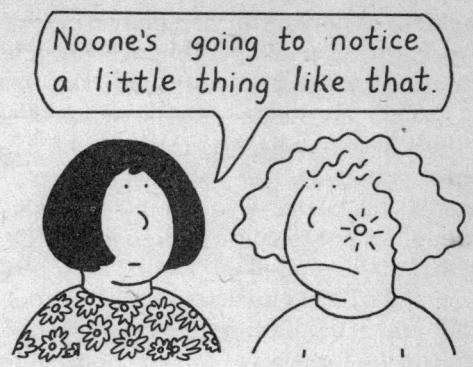

While those of us who have one spot, call it a 'spot' and others with three spots call theirs 'acne', spots and acne are really the same thing. People who regularly have several spots on the go are, however, usually more concerned about their skin than the lucky person who gets one spot a year.

Unfortunately, acne has until now been seen as just a 'skin complaint' – usually by adults who have forgotten what it feels like to look in the mirror three hours before a party, only to find a big red zit growing smack in the middle of their forehead. Telling you not to worry because 'you'll outgrow acne in a couple of years' and that anyway, 'other people won't notice it half as much as you', may be true, but it isn't exactly what you want to hear at the time.

Almost everyone gets acne to some degree, especially during their teenage years. By the way, one study found that, even in their fifties, 8 per cent of women and 6 per cent of men had some acne, and eight-year-olds can have a mild form of this, too.

There is a lot of information around on what you should or should not do about spots, but you can do something and it is important to learn about how to tackle your spots as soon as possible, for at least two reasons.
- To prevent scarring, pitting and discoloration of your skin in the long term.
- So you'll be less tempted to wear a mask when you go out.

The problem is that most of the spot creams, soaps, face scrubs and medicated cleansers and pads that are advertised as 'clearing

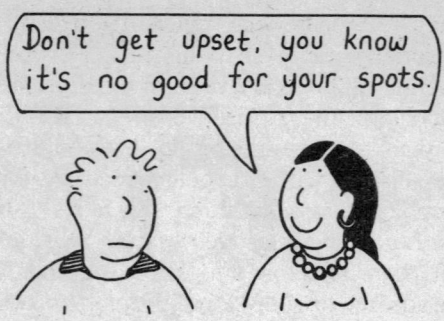

spots simply do not work. There are also a lot of ridiculous myths about the causes of spots.

Causes

Acne usually affects your face, back, chest and upper arms, and is often described as *mild, moderate* or *severe*. This depends on the number and size of your spots and how often you get them. If you want to control your acne, it is certainly worth spending a few minutes trying to understand exactly how spots are formed.

As you enter your teenage years, the level of the male hormone *testosterone*, which circulates around the bloodstream, rises. While both boys and girls need testosterone in order to develop into fully grown adults, boys have much more of this hormone. This is why boys tend to have more severe acne than girls. The rising levels of testosterone cause the oil glands beneath your skin to grow bigger and to produce much more oil. However, some people's oil glands over-react to this hormone, and it is this over-sensitivity that produces a greater number of blackheads and spots. Such 'bad luck' is inherited from your parents or grandparents in the same way as skin colour, eye colour and height, so acne may show up sooner or later no matter what you do or don't do. It is the areas with the most oil glands which are more likely to have acne. For example, while there are about 320 oil glands per square centimetre on your forehead, there are none on your palms or the soles of your feet.

The oil glands lie deep beneath the skin like an oil well and they pump oil up through your pores to the surface of your skin – this is like an oil pipeline. This oil is a natural moisturiser; if you didn't have any, you'd look like a dried prune by the time you were fourteen and your skin would be so dry you'd be in constant agony. The pore is lined with skin cells which are constantly being renewed. Normally they work their way to the surface and are washed away. But sometimes this system fails, and these cells combine with the rising oil and stick together, blocking the pipeline to the surface of your skin. The 'plug' of skin cells and oil which forms at the top of the pore is the all too familiar blackhead. The black colour of the blackhead is **not** caused by dirt; it is a natural reaction to the dried oil and skin cells being exposed to sunlight and air. So advertisements which sell soaps and cleaners 'to remove the dirt that causes blackheads' **are wrong**.

Most blackheads never develop into spots, probably because they do not block the pore completely. However, if the pore does become completely blocked then this means trouble, because the

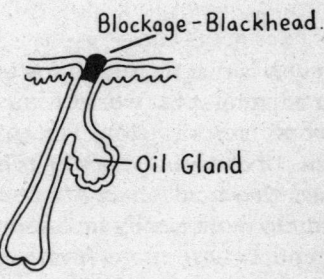

oil gland will still continue to pump oil up towards the plug. As this oil can't reach the surface, it creates a lot of pressure beneath the skin. Because of the increased pressure, the normal bacteria which live in the pore become over-active and change the trapped oil into irritating chemicals which inflame and damage the wall of the pore and invade the surrounding tissue. This is what causes the red swelling and the pain – the much hated spot. The more serious and the deeper this inflammation is, the more likely it is to turn into a *boil* and leave permanent scars and pits. Squeezing a spot that is not ready, or squeezing it in the wrong way, can

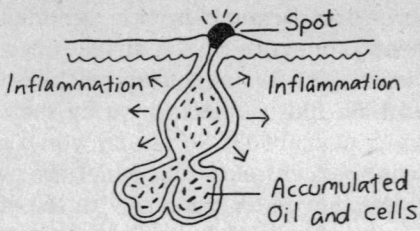

backfire by forcing the pus to explode downwards deep into the surrounding tissue, instead of upwards on to the surface of your skin. This is also likely to cause boils and bad scarring and pitting. So as you can see, spots are generally caused by what goes on beneath your skin, not on the surface.

Myths

There are many myths surrounding the causes of spots. Some of these myths help advertisers to sell you their useless remedies – at great expense to you, of course.

Foods

The most popular myth is that the foods you eat will either cause spots, or make your existing spots worse. Chocolate has long been considered the worst culprit. However, experiments where people had to eat lots of chocolate for weeks on end showed that this had no effect! Another food fallacy is that eating oily or greasy foods will make your skin more oily or cause more spots. So the oil in your chips is not about to travel from your stomach to your pores making your skin greasy and causing spots.

These foods do cause other problems though. Chocolate is basically melted fat, sugar and caffeine and its only function – apart from tasting good – is to rot your teeth, mess up your blood sugar levels and increase your chances of getting heart disease. Both chocolate and oily chips can also make you fat. The point is, that it is vital to follow a well-balanced, healthy diet in order to look and feel your best, and to help prevent a wide variety of illnesses, including cancer. Acne, however, is not a 'disease' which is either caused or cured by what you eat.

For example, the most recent idea is that eating organic 'whole foods' and fresh fruits and vegetables without additives will make all the difference to your spots. This is an excellent idea for your general health, although it is unlikely to be the answer to your spots. For more information on healthy eating, turn to Chapter 5.

Germs
Because spots contain pus, advertisers lead us to believe that they are caused by germs, or bacteria, which lurk on the surface of the skin. In fact, the bacteria involved in forming a spot are the normal kind which live in the pore anyway. Acne is **not** caused by bacteria on the skin; it is **not** an infection from bacteria invading your body; it does **not** spread from one area of your skin to another, nor from one person to another (by touching or using the same towel, for example). In rare cases it is possible for a spot which has already formed to become infected by harmful bacteria when it turns into a large boil; however, the original spot was not caused by external bacteria.

Not Washing Your Face Well Enough
Many people (and advertisers) say that 'you must keep your skin scrupulously clean, because dirt, grease, germs, toxins and pollutants build up on the skin, clogging pores and causing spots'. However, spots and blackheads are not caused by dirt and so, as many of you have already discovered, washing your face seven times a day is no better than washing it twice a day – in fact it can make it worse. So-called 'medicated' soaps and cleansers are a waste of money, as the medication just rinses away. Facial scrubs with rough particles such as ground peach stones are no better than a flannel and can actually make matters worse by irritating the skin and pores. It's very much the same as using scouring powder to polish your best silver.

'Zapping' Your Existing Spots
If you already have a spot, there is nothing you can buy to 'attack' it and make it go away. You will either have to hope that it develops a large white head so you can squeeze it properly, or else wait until it goes away naturally. Advertisements which show zits being 'blown away' or eradicated by 'high-powered' spot creams or medicated pencils just aren't true.

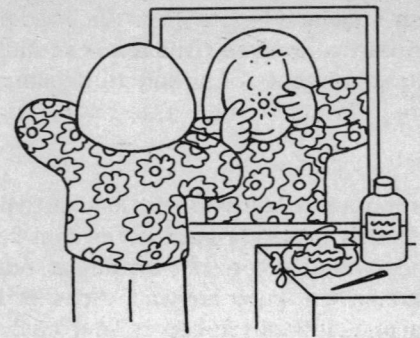

What Makes Acne Worse?

Menstrual Cycle

Girls' acne often appears or gets worse from seven to fourteen days before their monthly period arrives. This is due to the hormonal changes that occur at this time. Girls often crave chocolate during this time of the month, but if anything it is the hormonal changes, not the chocolate, that are responsible for the spots. Some older girls may find that contraceptive pills which only contain the hormone *progesterone* (the 'mini pill') can also aggravate acne.

Stress

Stress and worry can have a powerful effect on the balance between various hormones. For example, stress increases the amount of the stress hormones *cortisol* and *adrenaline* produced in your body. So if you are upset, your hormones can then be upset – and in some people, acne may flare up. Stress also makes many people crave chocolate, but again, it is probably the stress not the chocolate which causes the spots.

Heat and Humidity
Hot humid climates – even in Britain! – can make acne worse, because sweating increases oil production. Saunas can have the same effect.

Greasy Hair and Skin Products
Oil-based make-ups and hairdressings, moisturising creams and lubricating lotions can block your pores and prevent oil from reaching the skin's surface naturally. If you insist on wearing make-up, make sure it is water-based and oil-free. Try not to wear your hair down on your face in order to keep natural scalp oils off your skin. Scientists in America believe that some of the acne in black people is caused by pomade hair creams which can spread from the scalp to the face. Such hair creams and other products contain cocoa butter or coconut butter which are considered very *comedogenic* – in other words they are likely to cause blackheads to form. Certain suntan lotions can also cause problems (see Chapter 2).

Cosmetics
Certain cosmetics can irritate or block the lining of the pore and can cause or aggravate acne. However, because the ingredients in cosmetics change so frequently – and in many cases the ingredients are not even listed on the product label – it really isn't possible to provide you with a complete list of chemicals to avoid. But there are some major culprits, such as *isopropyl myristate, acetylated lanolin alcohol, lauric acid* and *laureth-4* which are highly comedogenic. Watch out for high-tech terms which are irrelevant. 'Hypoallergenic' means that the make-up is less likely to cause an allergic reaction, not that it will not cause blackheads. Many make-ups now use the term 'medicated'. This is also no guarantee that they will not cause blackheads, and besides, as spots are not caused by germs lurking on the surface of the skin, such 'medication' is useless. There are some good, inexpensive make-ups available which are better, not because they are 'medicated' but because they are simply water-based and oil-free. You will probably find more non-comedogenic cosmetics coming on the market as time goes by, so look out for them and ask your chemist.

16 SPOTS

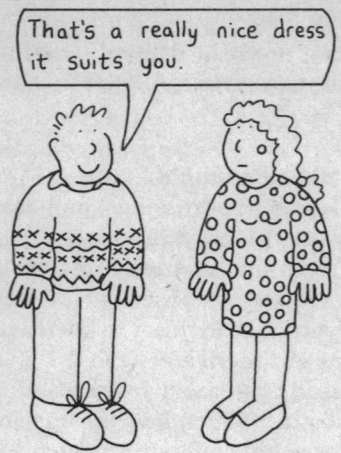

Clothing
Clothing made of natural fibres lets perspiration evaporate naturally, which is better for your skin. And while exercise is a must, it does cause you to sweat heavily, so ensure that you don't wear tight-fitting non-absorbent clothing or sweatbands made out of artificial fibres such as polyester or nylon.

The Right Way to Remove Blackheads and Squeeze Spots

As we discussed earlier, squeezing blackheads or spots in the wrong way can backfire, leaving you with boils and worse scarring than if you did nothing. While many doctors would like to tie your hands behind your back, the reality is that most of you are going to pick and squeeze no matter what you're told, so if you must do it, it is better to do it the right way.

Blackheads
Buy a *comedone spoon* from a chemist. Soften the area first by covering it with a warm wet flannel for about ten minutes. Aim the hole of the spoon directly over your target and press gently but firmly, not using too much force.

Spots
Never squeeze a spot unless it is 'ripe' – having a distinct white head on it. Wash your hands first and then, using a sterilized sharp needle, puncture and tear off the top of the white head. Next, use the tips of two fingers to press gently downwards, to get out the pus. Do not 'pinch' the spot and don't keep on pressing so as to force blood out or you may cause a scar, although the spot may bleed naturally anyway. Wash your hands and and clean the area around the spot with a mild antiseptic, which your chemist can advise you on.

How to Control Acne

There is nothing you can do to 'cure' acne once and for all, but you can keep it at bay until your oil glands settle down. Treatments must be continued as part of your everyday routine, often for years. This will prevent further spots from forming.

Washing
Use a mild soap which does not contain any moisturisers or perfume. The best soaps are often the cheapest – supermarket or chemists' own brands. If you have sensitive skin, ask your chemist or doctor for a *pH balanced* soap. If necessary, put a small amount of non-greasy moisturiser on any dry patches on your skin. You don't need to wash your face more than two or three times a day and don't use a flannel, as it is rough and can irritate the skin, and may well end up inflaming your pores.

Make-Up
Do not cover your skin with make-up more often than is necessary. Use it lightly and ensure it is water-based and oil-free or non-comedogenic.

Suntanning and Sun Lamps
Suntans tend to disguise acne but the risks of long-term skin damage which can lead to skin cancer are **not** worth the benefits (see Chapter 2). Suntanning may also interfere with the actions of some acne medicines.

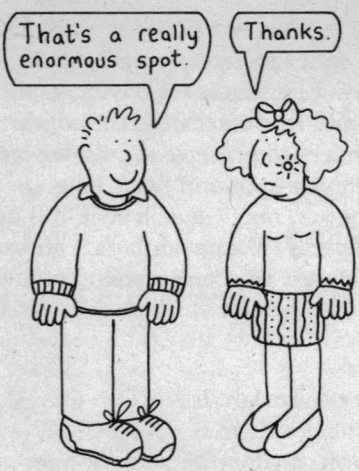

Spot Creams

Most spot products are a waste of money so think very carefully before you spend any money on them.

For mild acne, however, products which contain the chemical *benzoyl peroxide* may be helpful. This substance encourages dead skin cells to be discarded so that the pore openings remain clear. It will also reduce the amount of bacteria in your pores. Three strengths are available: 2.5, 5 and 10 per cent. Benzoyl peroxide is also prepared in different bases for different skin types. For example, while an *acetone* base may be suitable for darker, oily skin, a water or cream base may be better for fair, dry skin.

This chemical can make your skin go red. While this reaction should lessen after a while, fair-skinned people should start on the lowest strength and may at first need to apply it less often than the instructions say. Some people are allergic to it, so if you react strongly, stop using it.

You must apply benzoyl peroxide to the entire area prone to spots – not just to individual spots. Spot 'pencils' containing benzoyl peroxide are a complete waste of money and so are the benzoyl washes. People using benzoyl peroxide may find that their acne gets worse for a short time before it improves. If you use it on your back, chest or arms during the day, remember that it bleaches clothing, so wear an undershirt you don't care much about. Some of the lesser known brands behind the chemist's counter may be better or cheaper than the ones which are heavily advertised so ask the chemist for advice. If you are under sixteen you may be eligible for a free NHS prescription from your doctor. Discuss the type of product you need with your doctor and your chemist.

Prescription-Only Treatments

If the self-help measures aren't satisfactory, then your GP has a range of more powerful treatments available. You must realize, of course, that they will have to use their own judgement in deciding how to treat your acne. What is appropriate for someone else may be unsuitable for your skin. If you don't feel confident enough to ask your GP for help, then take your parents or an older brother or sister with you. Remember acne should be taken seriously and you have a **right** to ask for your doctor's help. You should **not** feel that you are wasting their time. They are there to help you and most will be sympathetic. Explain that you have a problem which is making you miserable. You are aware of some of the treatments around and need their help.

Whatever they suggest, you must realize that it takes some time for any treatment to work – sometimes several months. Unfortunately many people give up after only a few weeks and lose hope. **Do not give up.** Adverts which promise quick results don't work. Again, see your GP if you're not happy with the results of the treatment – they want to know so they can help you more effectively.

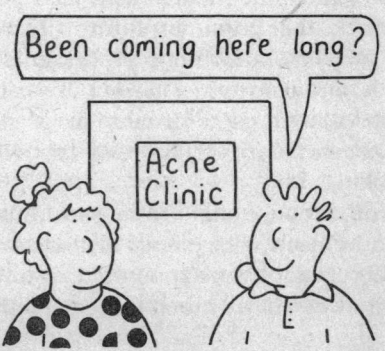

If your acne does prove particularly difficult to treat, your GP may refer you to a skin specialist, a *dermatologist*, who will be able to suggest new treatments.

Some of the treatments you may be offered are explained below.

Topical Antibiotics

These are lotions or solutions which you put directly on your skin. They work by preventing the normal bacteria in your pores from getting out of hand. They are very effective against mild or moderate acne. There are two bases available, one is a liquid alcohol solution and the other is a lotion for sensitive skin.

Antibiotic Tablets

For moderate to severe acne, the doctor may prescribe antibiotics. *Tetracyclines* are the most well known of these tablets, but they do produce side-effects in some people, such as stained teeth, thrush of the digestive system or vagina, and diarrhoea. Discuss this carefully with your GP first. If you do start taking antibiotic tablets and you wish to stop, then ask your GP and slowly reduce the amount of tablets you take. Never stop suddenly, as your acne may react terribly and become much worse very quickly.

Tretinoin

Tretinoin is a mild acid which you put on your skin once a day. It works by gradually loosening the plugs which may be blocking some of the pores, and continues to keep them clear by ensuring that the skin cells which line the inside of your pores do not stick together and block the pores in future. This prevents both blackheads and spots from forming. Tretinoin is available under the name 'Retin-A' and comes in a variety of strengths and bases. For example, the lotion is used for large areas such as the back, the gel is for darker and more oily types of skin, while the cream is for fairer, drier skin.

Tretinoin will often cause slight redness and flaking of the skin and may need to be used with plenty of moisturisers. You must protect your skin from over-exposure to sunlight and avoid sunlamps as your skin will be much more sensitive to ultraviolet light.

Female Hormone (Oestrogen) Tablets

These are only prescribed for girls and are sometimes used when other methods have failed. They reduce the size of the oil glands. Since the amount of oil produced is less when the glands are smaller, there is less chance of spots developing. Oestrogens may have unwanted side-effects, however. Sometimes a special form of contraceptive pill which contains less oestrogen and an *anti-testosterone* substance is used not as a contraceptive but as a treatment. Discuss this with your GP as you need to consider this option carefully.

Isotretinoin Tablets

Only used in cases of severe acne which have not responded to other types of treatment, these can only be prescribed by a consultant. Isotretinoin dramatically reduces the amount of oil produced by the oil glands, changes the normal bacteria in the pores, and also encourages the removal of dead skin cells, thereby unblocking the pores. As a result, they are extremely effective. The medicine is taken for three to four months only and you will be monitored regularly to check the side-effects, which should be clearly explained to you before hand.

Direct Corticosteroid Injection

If you have a particularly large boil (cyst), a direct injection can be very beneficial in reducing the inflammation. Dermatologists may use this method if you frequently get cysts which could leave scars.

Summing Up

As you can see, there is plenty that can be done for your acne, and fortunately nowadays everyone can be helped. There is one final point worth mentioning. Most people with spots spend time examining their skin closely in front of a mirror, often under bright light. This gives you a false idea of how noticeable your spots are. By focusing your attention on every lump and blackhead, you can easily exaggerate how bad your skin really looks – and make yourself unnecessarily miserable. So keep busy and enjoy yourself while your treatments take effect.

For further support and advice on acne send a stamped addressed envelope to:

The Acne Support Group, 16 DuFour's Place, Broadwick Street, London, W1V 1FE.

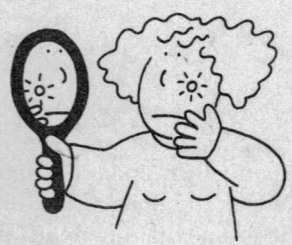

Chapter 2
Suntanning

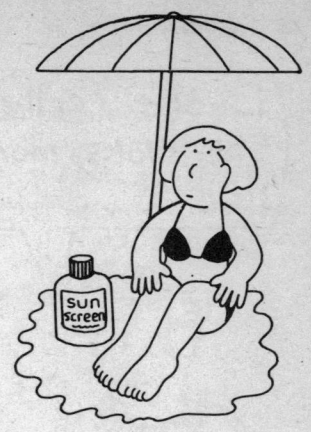

The way you feel about your acne today is the way you will feel about having a wrinkled, alligator-skinned face when you are thirty-five. Now is the time to find out what too much sun can do to your skin so that you can take the simple and sensible precautions which will help you avoid any problems.

Years ago, a suntan was a sign of being of a lower social class because you had to work under direct sunlight outdoors in the fields or on the roads for a living. The posher you were, the less likely you were to have to be outdoors in strong sunlight, and so pale ivory skin was associated with being upper class or aristocratic, especially for women.

Over the past forty years all this has changed. People from all backgrounds wanted to look tanned like the Hollywood movie stars. Foreign package holidays in sunny climates became available to millions of families and so did sunlamps and sunbeds – now everyone could look like a star.

Photodamage

However, our long-term love affair with the suntan is coming to an end. Even the world's most famous models have now stopped tanning themselves, and those who do need to look tanned often use fake self-tanning creams for their photo sessions. The same goes for many famous actors and actresses – even those who appear in sunny Australian or American soap operas.

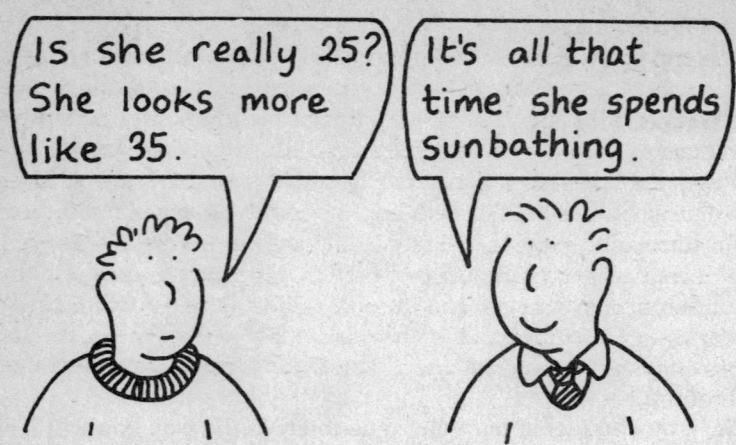

There are good reasons for this. While we all need small amounts of sunlight for our general good health, we now understand that too much direct sun is seriously bad for you. Those rich, dark Mediterranean tans you used to envy now indicate skin that had been damaged by the sun's rays. The term used to describe the damage to the skin caused by the sun is *photodamage* and it is caused by not protecting yourself adequately from too much sun.

Up to 90 per cent of the skin's ageing is caused by being in the sun too much, making your skin wrinkled and dry. Models, actors and actresses cannot afford to have patchy, dry, leathery and wrinkled skin, or else their careers will be even shorter than they are already. And, if they are not careful, many young people will find that they end up with faces like dried prunes.

Not only that, but there is a world-wide epidemic of skin cancers, at least 75 per cent of which could probably be prevented if people used adequate protection against the sun's rays during the first eighteen years of their life. Most people get 50 per cent of their lifetime's exposure to the sun by the time they are eighteen, and some scientists suspect that while you are growing up, your skin is developing and is particularly vulnerable to permanent cancerous changes. While we used to think of skin cancers as being a disease of older people, the age is dropping.

The Ozone Layer

One important factor in the early ageing of skin and the increase in skin cancer is the change in the earth's atmosphere. Ozone, which surrounds the earth, filters out much of the sun's ultraviolet rays (radiation) which can damage the skin. You know about the enormous holes that have developed in the earth's ozone layer because of pollution. These holes have allowed larger amounts of this ultraviolet radiation to reach us than ever before. For every 1 per cent loss in the ozone layer there is a 3 per cent increase in the number of skin cancers, and Europe has lost between 8 and 20 per cent of its ozone layer over the past twelve years (the degree of loss changes with the weather). This means that we must be more careful than ever.

What Causes the Damage?

Ultraviolet radiation is invisible rays of sunlight which are divided into three types: UVA, UVB and UVC. UVA causes skin ageing, tanning and sometimes burning. This type of radiation is long wavelength and penetrates deep into the skin, contributing to skin cancer in the long run. UVB is shorter wavelength, penetrating less deeply into the skin. But it is the main cause of suntan, sunburn and skin cancers. UVC is absorbed by the atmosphere and doesn't reach the earth's surface.

When your skin is exposed to the sun, it tries to protect itself by becoming thicker and producing the brown tanning pigment called *melanin* which absorbs UV rays before they cause more damage. This is what gives you a suntan.

Some people naturally have less melanin in their skins and therefore burn far more easily than others. Those with blonde or red hair, blue eyes and very fair skin usually burn far more quickly than darker-skinned, brown-eyed brunettes, for example. Black people and other dark-skinned people get their natural skin colour from the high amount of melanin that occurs naturally in their skin. These people are therefore heavily protected from UV rays all the time. They rarely get skin cancers from sunlight and their skin is less likely to age early because of photodamage. In the past, countries closer to the North Pole were populated by fairer-

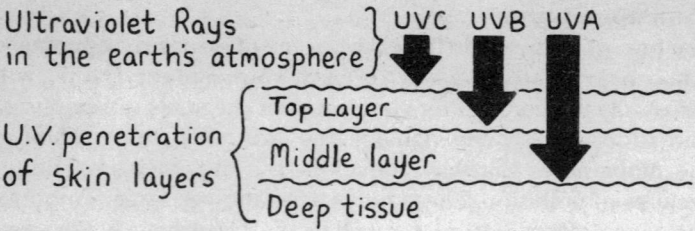

skinned people, and countries closer to the equator were populated by darker-skinned people. Different races developed to cope with the amount of sunlight they were exposed to in their environment. Even today, for example, Iceland, which is 65 degrees north of the equator, is full of pale-skinned people, while Kenya, which is on the equator, is mainly populated by black-skinned people. So, we can begin to see that fair-skinned British people were really not designed to tolerate lots of intense sunlight. Holidays to hot sunny climates are a shock to British skin and put a huge and sudden strain on its ability to protect itself.

In people who are not dark skinned to start with but who develop and maintain a tan so they look more brown, being exposed to UV rays destroys the elastic fibres in the skin which causes it to sag and wrinkle, and damages the fine blood vessels and the skin's immune system. Even though people who tan easily may seem to be less likely to get skin cancer, they still need to be protected from the sun's ultraviolet rays.

There Is No Such Thing as a Safe Tan

A suntan is a sign that your skin has been damaged and is trying to protect itself from any more harm. A tan is damaging whether you tan quickly and easily or do it very slowly over several weeks. Although a suntan may protect you against sunburn (which is even more damaging), it is still a sign that you are taking in and storing the effects of harmful radiation – it all adds up. Redness is not the only sign of sun damage. Microscopic changes to the skin (which can only be detected in the laboratory) occur even when you prevent a sunburn.

It is important to realize that every exposure to UV rays is stored in our skin and the effects add up over time whether we burn or not. Think of your skin as a bottle into which you slowly pour sun exposure, several minutes or a couple of hours at a time. Over time, as the bottle fills, the damage adds up and as it nears the top, skin cancer can result. By limiting our exposure, we can try to ensure it never reaches the top. This means avoiding sunburn and accepting less of a tan as well as following the advice below.

A sunburn is a more extreme degree of damage than a suntan. In fact, people who have had three or more bad sunburns with blisters before they reach eighteen appear to be more likely to get malignant melanoma, the most serious form of skin cancer. Do not try to get a 'quick' tan.

Sunbeds Are Not Safer

Sunbeds, sunlamps and solariums give out mostly UVA radiation. This is less likely to cause an immediate sunburn than UVB radiation so people assume it must be safer. This is not true, and because the brown colour takes longer to show up from UVA exposure, some sunbeds give out **ten times** the UVA radiation that sunlight has in order to produce a so-called 'quick tan'. UVA will penetrate more deeply into the skin and will age it. It may also damage the blood vessels and prevent the immune system from protecting your skin. It will also 'sensitize' the skin, which allows sunlight to cause skin cancers more easily, so using a sunbed to prepare your skin for the real sun outdoors increases your risk of skin cancer and premature ageing even more. So do not combine the two.

Don't Believe All the Adverts

Sunscreens are an essential part of protecting your skin from the sun, as we will discuss later, but when you are buying, look for hard facts and be very sceptical about the claims that some advertisers make about their products.

Advertisers are trying to make you buy their product rather than someone else's, so they can be guilty of making extravagant claims. They often try to sell you their suntan lotions by giving the impression that suntans are healthier and make you fitter. They confuse the fact that everyone needs small regular doses of daylight with the idea that we will actually benefit from a suntan. Of course they say that you can 'tan safely' by using their suntan lotions to reduce the amount of UV rays you receive. They feel that by 'tanning gradually' (using their products) you will be 'tanning safely'. They choose their words very carefully when they come out with statements like: 'The experts tell us that sunshine is good for our health, and when it comes to feeling healthier, fitter and happier – nothing can beat a lovely golden tan!'

Notice two things:

1 The words imply, without actually saying it, that the so-called experts actually prefer us to have a tan. Rubbish! Dermatologists would prefer us not to have a suntan.

2 They are careful to say that a suntan makes us **feel** healthier and fitter not that it actually does make us healthier and fitter. This is because it doesn't and they know it.

Of course, they won't be there holding your hand in ten years time when your face looks like the inside of a leather boot. No, instead they'll be trying to sell you anti-wrinkle creams to undo all the damage!

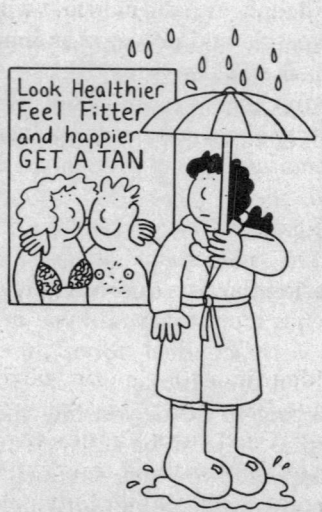

Suntans and Acne

As we discussed earlier, a suntan will do nothing more than help to disguise spots temporarily. However, many of the acne treatments make your skin much more sensitive to UV rays (*photosensitive*). In other words, you can burn very easily, which will no doubt make you even more unhappy when you look in the mirror. Many suntan lotions can aggravate acne. If you have oily skin or acne, try sunscreens in a clear gel or lotion. You should use more oily sunscreens if you need a moisturiser. You'll probably have to experiment a bit.

Photoprotection

Fortunately, modern sunscreens and sunblocks can give you very effective protection against the sun. You won't need to avoid sunshine or refuse to go on holiday abroad, just take sensible precautions when you are out in the sun.

Remember that you must take precautions no matter what you are doing. Activities such as sitting at a football match, riding your bike, sightseeing on holiday or skateboarding expose you to just as much sun as lying on a beach.

Beware, too, of hot but cloudy days. You can get a sunburn even on a cloudy day. In fact, without the intensity of heat to warn you, you may be even more likely to burn.

Even if you have decided that you want to get a suntan anyway, it is still worth reading on to learn how to make it 'less unsafe'.

Timing Your Exposure
There is more UV radiation between 10.00 a.m. and 3.00 p.m. when the sun is strongest, so cover up during these hours and tan earlier or later if you must. Remember, tan slowly.

Clothing
Clothing and a wide-brimmed hat are extremely effective at screening out UV rays. Blue denim, for example, has an SPF (*sun protection factor*) of 1000! Cotton fabrics are best. So if you are out in the sun and cannot bear to be constantly greasing yourself up with sunscreens, cover up with clothing.

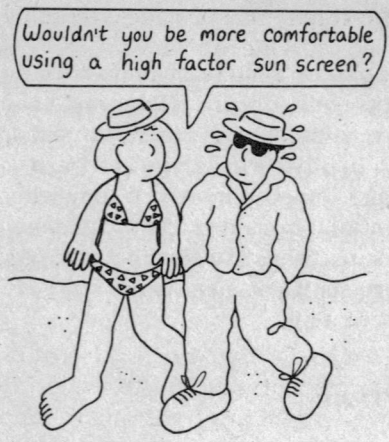

The Sun Protection Factor

When you buy a sunscreen, the SPF number will tell you how long you can stay in the sun before you burn. For example, a sunscreen with an SPF of 15 would allow you to stay in the sun without burning for fifteen times longer, on average, than if you didn't use the sunscreen. So if you're fair-skinned and fair-haired and would normally burn in ten minutes, a sunscreen with SPF 15 would allow you 150 minutes before you burn. Don't go out of your way to discover how long it takes you to burn without a sunscreen – just assume you burn easily, in six to ten minutes. Those with darker hair, brown eyes and a more olive skin may take longer to roast, perhaps fifteen to twenty minutes. Asians can tolerate more sun than most light-skinned people, and black people have the best protection. Therefore people who burn more easily need a higher SPF number. Remember that any examples are average, so always err on the side of caution.

UVA Protection

Unfortunately, the SPF rating only tells you how much protection you'll get from UVB rays. So two sunscreens with the same SPF number can offer very different protection against UVA rays. An SPF 15 may be excellent protection from UVB rays but may provide little protection from the UVA rays, so when you choose a sunscreen, make sure it also provides adequate UVA protection. There is, as yet, no separate SPF number for UVA. However, some shops are providing a star-rating which will give you a general idea of whether you will get the same level of protection from UVA and UVB when you buy a particular SPF. We really need clear labelling laws to ensure that we know exactly what protection we are getting.

If you are going to be out in the sun and you don't care whether you tan or not, then use at least SPF 20 with high UVA protection. For hotter, sunnier climates, use at least an SPF 30 with high UVA protection.

If you want a suntan but you want to limit the amount of damage and reduce your risk of skin cancer, then find the right SPF number for your skin type, again with high UVA protection. Advertisers and chemists may have their own charts which recommend lower SPF numbers, but as it is better to be safe than sorry, ignore them.

The chart on page 32 takes into account how many hours you expect to be in the sun on a particular day and the climate you are going to be in:

AREA 1: Countries in the UK and Northern Europe
AREA 2: Hotter, sunnier places such as the Mediterranean or Florida
AREA 3: The hottest, sunniest places closer to the equator like Kenya, Singapore and Northern Australia

By the way, if you ski, you should use a higher SPF as higher altitudes expose you to much more UV radiation.

Extra Points to Remember

- Products claiming to be *waterproof* should protect you at their SPF level even after you spend eighty minutes in the water. Those products claiming to be *water-resistant* are only good for about forty minutes. If you are going swimming or playing sports that make you sweat heavily then remember this difference.

- People often apply only **half** the amount of sunscreen that they should. This means that a factor 15 could drop to a factor 8. Use plenty! Also apply it frequently – a single dose won't remain effective for long periods.

Choosing Your Sun Protection Factor

Skin Type

Expected Time in Sun Each Day	Extremely Sun-Sensitive: Never Tans, Always Burns			Sun-Sensitive: Tans Slowly, Burns Easily			Fair Complexion: Tans Gradually, Usually Burns First			Medium Complexion: Tans Well, Sometimes Burns			Dark Complexion: Tans Easily, Rarely Burns		
Less than 1 hour	SPF 15	SPF 15	SPF 20	SPF 8	SPF 8	SPF 12	SPF 6	SPF 6	SPF 8	SPF 4	SPF 4	SPF 6	SPF 2	SPF 2	SPF 4
1-2 hours	SPF 25	SPF 25	SPF 30	SPF 12	SPF 15	SPF 20	SPF 8	SPF 8	SPF 12	SPF 6	SPF 6	SPF 10	SPF 4	SPF 4	SPF 6
2-3 hours	SPF 30	SPF 30	SPF 30+	SPF 20	SPF 25	SPF 30	SPF 12	SPF 15	SPF 20	SPF 6	SPF 8	SPF 12	SPF 4	SPF 6	SPF 10
3-4 hours	SPF 30	SPF 30	SPF 30+	SPF 25	SPF 30	SPF 30+	SPF 20	SPF 25	SPF 30	SPF 10	SPF 15	SPF 20	SPF 6	SPF 8	SPF 12
5-6 hours	SPF 30	SPF 30+	SPF 30+	SPF 30	SPF 30	SPF 30+	SPF 25	SPF 25	SPF 30+	SPF 20	SPF 25	SPF 30	SPF 12	SPF 15	SPF 20
Over 6 hours	SPF 30	SPF 30+	SPF 30+	SPF 30	SPF 30+	SPF 30+	SPF 25	SPF 30+	SPF 30+	SPF 25	SPF 30	SPF 30+	SPF 20	SPF 25	SPF 30
	1	2	3	1	2	3	1	2	3	1	2	3	1	2	3

Climate of Country

SUNTANNING 33

- If you are fair-skinned and will be outside all day, use a factor 30 or more. However, some of the higher SPF formulae may irritate your skin because their chemicals are so concentrated. In this case, simply apply a lower SPF sunscreen more frequently than normal – or cover up with clothes.

- Try to apply your sunscreen at least thirty to forty-five minutes before you are exposed to the sun. This allows the active ingredients to become more firmly attached to the skin.

- Just because your skin isn't turning red while you're in the sun doesn't mean you're not burning. A sunburn is most noticeable from between six to twenty-four hours **after** being in the sun. The same goes for a suntan.

- A session under a sunbed or in heavy sunshine can cause a very serious reaction if you're taking medications such as antibiotics, antihistamines, oral contraceptives or hormone tablets. Always ask your GP or chemist about the interaction between the medication you're using and UV rays.

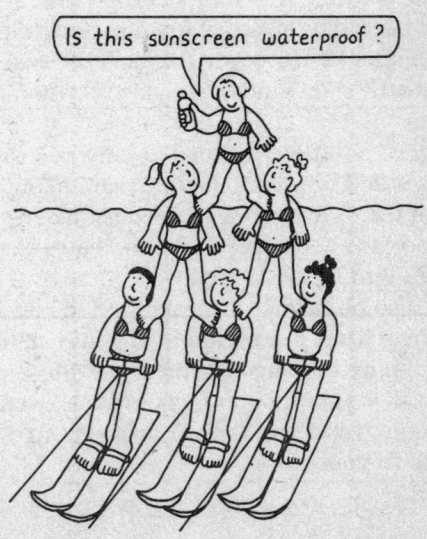

- After you have been in the sun, always smooth on plenty of moisturiser.

- When you buy sunscreens, you are often paying for the name and the company's advertising programme. Select a sunscreen made by a reliable company with the SPF and UVA protection you require, not because it has a 'designer' name on the bottle.

Shades

Sunglasses are going to become even more popular. This is not because they're trendy but because there is mounting evidence that bright sunlight can, over time, cause permanent damage to the lens and the retina of the eye. While Britain is not exactly the sunniest country to live in, the changing ozone layer again makes this an important issue to think about. More people are exposed to bright sunlight through sailing, skiing and trips to sunny climates as well. Remember sand, snow and water make sunlight even stronger by reflecting it back at you.

The need to protect our eyes from intense light might, on the surface, seem to conflict with our need to take in a sufficient amount of light each day in order for our body clocks to work normally (see Chapter 8). However, this isn't the case. It's simply a matter of wearing the right kind of sunglasses when you're in very bright conditions.

First of all, there is little relationship between the colour and darkness of lenses and how well they can screen out UV rays. It is UVB in particular that is damaging to the lens. When you buy a pair of sunglasses, look for a 'tie tag' which indicates that the glasses meet British Standard BS2724 (1987).

There should also be further information indicating how much protection you're getting. For example, if you're going skiing you will need special-purpose lenses which provide greater protection. If in doubt ask your optician or chemist. Also ensure that the lenses are big enough and that they fit properly so that the lenses are close enough to your eyes.

Coping with Sunburn

So, you have ignored all this information and come in from the sun pink and sore. What do you do? From the point of view of immediate first aid, sunburn is the same as any other burn, so the first thing to do is to reduce the heat in the skin tissues. Bathe the area in cool water or lie in a cool bath for at least 10 minutes. Wear loose cotton clothing so that nothing rubs the sore skin, and smooth on a little calomine or similar lotion to ease the discomfort. Greasy products, like baby oil or 'after-sun' creams seal in heat, while so-called 'cooling lotions' containing menthol or camphor can end up causing worse irritation or allergic reactions. If the skin is seriously burnt or blistered, you may think about seeing your GP. Never break blisters, just leave the skin to heal gradually. Cover up, and don't expose the skin to the sun again until it is completely healed. Most important of all – don't do it again.

Summing Up

Your first eighteen years are critical in protecting your skin from sun damage which could lead to serious health problems in the future. If you don't believe me, all I can say is, 'Get well soon!'

Chapter 3
Weight and
Body Shape

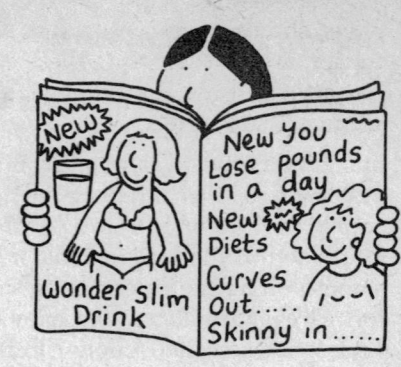

The Beautiful People Con

This section applies mainly to the girls, but it concerns and interests both boys and girls.

There is an enormous industry out there that **wants** you to be unhappy with your weight and body shape. They have been highly successful – because if you were satisfied with your weight you probably wouldn't be reading this chapter!

The diet industry which sells 'slimming aids', 'lean' foods, books, magazines and runs slimming centres is worth about £21 billion a year. If you were happy with your weight they would be out of business. Worse than the diet industry are womens' magazines, television programmes and adverts.

Womens' magazines would like you to think of them as your friends – sharing their ideas, concerns, news and interests with you. However, they are certainly **not** your friends! They are a business that has to sell you their magazines and the products advertised within the magazines in order to make a profit. They are contaminated by the beauty and fashion industry – and this is how it works.

That Feel-Good Factor
If you pick up any magazine, you'll notice that almost every girl photographed is abnormally slim with a beautiful face. By the way, they always make sure that a skinny body is connected to a beautiful face. This helps give you the impression that it is actually the skinny body that is the key to being attractive. After all, we're

never shown a girl with a slim figure and a mush like a pit bull terrier, are we? By using these unnatural photos, they can draw our attention to their articles and advertisements. Even articles about peanut butter which have no relationship whatsoever with slim bodies, appear with photos of abnormally slender girls with beautiful faces. Photos of girls modelling clothes are a con, because what you don't see are the bulldog clips holding the clothing together at the back to give the impression of a perfect fit. Skinny girls are used because the clothes themselves are easier to photograph and sell.

That Feel-Bad Factor

If these photos make you feel less attractive and unhappy with your weight, then the editors and advertisers are happy, because you can buy their products, such as a new outfit, make-up and hair products, to make you feel more attractive – more like the girls in the photos. You may also be more likely to read their articles, which subconsciously you hope will bring you closer to their world of beautiful, slim, happy people! But after seeing hundreds or thousands of these girls in magazine photos and television adverts and programmes, you are more likely **not** to feel part of the world of beautiful, slim, happy people. In fact you will probably feel **less** satisfied with the way you look than when you started. You can then write to their problem page because, of course, this is also good for business! If people were satisfied with the way they looked they wouldn't spend as much on new ideas and new things to make themselves more attractive.

The real joke is that while the girls in the magazines and on the telly have unusually slim bodies and beautiful faces, the editors, writers and producers who constantly rub these images in your face certainly don't look like this themselves!

Scientists are now becoming very concerned about the effect that all these magazines and television pictures are having on the health of women. A recent report found that even girls as young as nine are now going on slimming diets so they can try and be as skinny as the models they admire in magazines and on television. This is particularly dangerous because so-called weight-loss diets **do not work** in the long run and can easily make you fatter. In fact, about 95 per cent of people who go on a diet end up the same weight or even bigger within a year. Young girls and teenagers who diet may prevent their bones from growing normally and they can also prevent their female hormones which make them look like girls (softer, smoother hair and skin, for example), from developing and working properly. Dieting also affects the chemicals in your brain and can make you depressed.

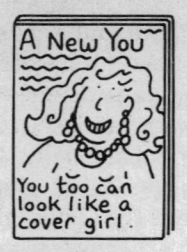

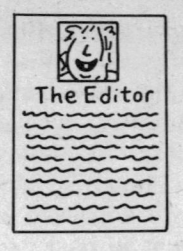

It's come to the point now, where one out of four women is on a 'slimming' diet and nine out of ten women are unhappy with their body shape. Things are a mess. And we now find that many of the **wrong** people are trying to lose weight for the **wrong** reasons using the **wrong** methods. There is a huge rise in the number of people with serious eating disorders. Dieting when you are young is linked with being eight times more likley to develop *anorexia* or *bulimia* – which are potentially fatal. Experts have continually warned the media that the constant display of images of so-called perfect bodies is contributing to these eating disorders. Unfortunately, the fact that anorexia can have fatal consequences still hasn't stopped these lovely friends of ours – the editors, advertisers and TV producers – from continuing to shove unrealistically slim models in your face to keep you feeling insecure about the way you look.

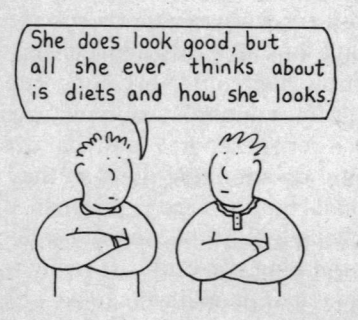

Why Are Models Slim?

A camera generally makes people look slightly heavier (about 5 kilos) than they really are. Therefore, when you see a model or an actress in a photo or on television, she is even skinnier in real life.

We like to think that they are so slim because they 'watch their weight' by 'dieting properly' and that if we had their self-control then we too could look as slim as them. **This is completely false!**

A recent study of modelling agencies in New York found that models are born with their thin body shape. In fact, models have very abnormal figures – they are in general 10 centimetres taller but weigh 2 kilos less than the average woman. They **do not** diet all the time and are far less likely to have anorexia than normal women!

In other words, no amount of dieting will give you that abnormal body look – you have to inherit it. Many Hollywood movie stars don't have this abnormal body shape and a skinnier model who looks similar to the famous actress will stand in for her in certain scenes so that you will think the star is slimmer than she really is!

My office is actually next door to a modelling agency in London so I showed this section on slim models to the women who own the agency. They fully agreed with what I wrote and added 'girls should not even attempt to be slim like our models, they should leave it to the professionals who are *born* that way. Magazine and television adverts which use our models are selling a fantasy, and girls should realize this'. Some of you are born with bigger bones or wider hips or more body fat and it's important to accept this because if you try to 'fight it out' with your own biology, your biology will win and you will lose!

You can't change your body shape the way you can change your hairstyle.

Are Slim Girls Really Happier?

No! In fact many of them are more miserable. Psychiatric hospitals are full of slender women – their slim figures do not protect them from severe depression or nervousness. Many ballet dancers, for instance, are terribly self-conscious and always worry about their weight, even though they are painfully thin. A large number have anorexia or bulimia and while they may look wonderful gliding across a stage, this does not by any means show that they are happy and confident people with lots of amazing boyfriends.

Are Slim Girls More Attractive to Boys?

Sadly, most girls believe that boys generally prefer girls with slim figures. But in fact, scientific studies have found that you are wrong! Boys actually find a variety of things attractive – your figure is only one of them. Unfortunately many of you girls wrongly assume that it is your weight that boys focus on. In reality, however, boys are 'turned on' by your smile, your hair, your face, your breasts, your eyes, your voice, your sense of humour. Even a girl's confidence – the way she 'carries' herself – has a big effect on boys. The ultra-slim model type who is self-conscious, always looking at her reflection in shop windows, can put boys off for two reasons:
- She doesn't seem very 'warm', and wouldn't be much fun.
- She may appear to be dissatisfied with her appearance in which case boys are influenced by this and may also think less of her appearance.

Many girls waste their time trying to 'hide' what they consider to be their 'chubby thighs' or their 'big bottom'. What they don't know is that boys can see right through all of that – they can tell what your body shape looks like no matter what you wear. Furthermore, boys actually **like** the fat on your hips, thighs and bottom, because they fancy what is **different** from them. Why on earth would they want you to have the same type of slim hips, thighs and bottom that they do? The fact that your shape is changing and becoming different from theirs is an important signal to them that you are a member of the opposite sex.

Young people do not necessarily grow at an even pace. When 'growth spurts' occur, this may change your shape or weight rather quickly. Sometimes you may grow wider first and taller second, or you may grow tall quickly but not fill in until afterwards. In any event, for girls, fat on hips, thighs and bottoms is normal, healthy and absolutely necessary to produce the hormones that make you look feminine.

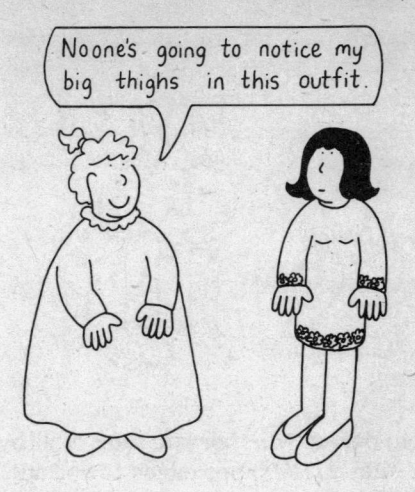

The point of the first part of this chapter is to **think** how you're being affected and conned by magazine and television images of unrealistically slim beautiful girls. These images are being pushed on to you for profit-motives alone. Push them back!

Do You Really Need to Lose Weight?

The whole idea of weight is a bit misleading and out of date. For example, as muscle weighs more than fat, a fit, slim girl who takes size 10 in clothes could find herself weighing more than an unfit girl who takes size 12. It's all down to *body composition* – how much of your body is made up of fat versus muscle and tissue. If a boy and a girl are exactly the same height and general size, the boy will weigh more than the girl; his hormones ensure that he has more muscle than her, while her hormones ensure she has more fat than him, especially on her hips, thighs and bottom. Muscle also requires more food, so boys generally need to eat more than girls. If that same boy and girl run a kilometre at the same speed, he will automatically burn up more calories.

42 WEIGHT AND BODY SHAPE

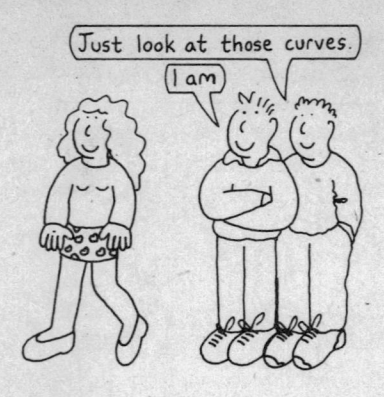

(Just look at those curves.)
(I am)

The best way to decide whether you are a healthy size is to find your *body mass index* [*(BMI)* See pages 44 and 45]. This is a more modern method than the old height and weight charts. If you find your weight falls between those entries given, you can easily estimate your approximate BMI which will fall between the two figures. Generally, for males, a healthy body mass is around 22 to 24. Over 28.5 is unhealthy and above 33 you are seriously unhealthy. For females, a healthy body mass is generally around 21 to 23. Over 27.5 becomes unhealthy and above 31.5 is seriously unhealthy.

Is Your Body Shape Healthy?

If you are a teenager or older and concerned about your body shape, there is a new way of checking whether it is healthy by finding your *waist to hip ratio (WHR)* on page 46. You will first need to measure your waist at the navel, then your hips at the greatest point around the bottom. A WHR greater than 1.0 for males and 0.8 for females indicates that you may be storing fat in the wrong places (deep inside the stomach). This could lead to certain problems later on. So, a male's waist shouldn't be larger than his hips, while a female's hips should be at least 20 per cent larger than her waist. For example, a girl with a 63 centimetre waist and 89 centimetre hips has a waist to hip ratio of 0.71. Since this is less than 0.8 it is healthy.

Girls, remember the fat on hips, thighs and bottoms is normal, attractive, healthy and necessary! If you have a healthy BMI and WHR then **leave well alone**.

If you are uncertain about your weight and shape, see your GP. If it does turn out that your BMI and WHR are unhealthy, then the worst thing you can do is go on a so-called 'weight loss diet' – they are rubbish.

What Dieting Can Do for You!

- Dieting makes your body slow down the rate at which it burns up your body fat. So when you decide to limit your diet and lose 5 kilos, your body becomes used to the new limited diet. Then if you increase the amount of food you eat again, even though you still eat **less** than you did before your diet, your body treats the increase as if it were extra and stores it as fat – so you gain back the weight!
- People who 'yo-yo' diet (losing weight quickly, only to regain it again) can damage their metabolism and will take longer each time to lose weight but will gain it back more quickly. The terrifying thing is that each time you gain the weight back, more of it will be fat and less of it will be muscle, and because muscle is so good at burning up calories, you are losing your best natural weight control aid, so you will instead end up more flubbery than when you started.
- Repeated yo-yo dieting is thought to damage your body in a way that increases your chances of heart disease.
- Because dieting is unnatural, it messes up your appetite control mechanism. This means that you'll be less able to control your hunger and tell when you're full, and you'll be more likely to binge. You will also be more likely to choose fattening foods when you go off the diet. All of this will simply make you fatter.
- If girls are interested in growing a beard and moustache, they may well have their wish – as staying below your natural healthy weight upsets your hormones and causes facial hair growth!

WEIGHT AND BODY SHAPE

Weight in pounds

Height in metres	100	105	110	115	120	125	130	135	140
1.83								18.2	19.1
1.80							18.2	18.8	19.7
1.78							18.6	19.2	20.2
1.75						18.6	19.3	19.9	20.9
1.73					18.4	19	19.7	20.4	21.4
1.70					19	19.7	20.4	21.1	22.1
1.68				18.4	19.5	20.2	20.9	21.6	22.7
1.65				19.1	20.2	20.9	21.7	22.4	23.5
1.63			18.1	18.8	19.6	20.7	21.4	22.2	23	24.1
1.60		18.7	19.5	20.3	21.5	22.3	23	23.8	25
1.58	18	19.2	20	20.8	22	22.8	23.6	24.4	25.6
1.55	18.7	20	20.8	21.6	22.9	23.7	24.6	25.4	26.6
1.53	19.2	20.5	21.4	22.2	23.5	24.3	25.2	26.1	27.3
1.50	20	21.3	22.2	23.1	24.4	25.3	26.2	27.1	28.4
1.48	20.5	21.9	22.8	23.7	25.1	26	26.9	27.8	29.2
	45	48	50	52	55	57	59	61	64

Weight in kilograms

Body Mass

WEIGHT AND BODY SHAPE 45

Weight in pounds

145	150	155	160	165	170	175	180	185	
19.7	20.3	20.9	21.5	22.4	23	23.6	24.5	25.1	6'
20.4	21	21.6	22.2	23.1	23.8	24.4	25.3	25.6	5'11"
20.8	21.5	22.1	22.7	23.7	24.3	24.9	25.9	26.5	5'10"
21.5	22.2	22.9	23.5	24.5	25.1	25.8	26.8	27.4	5'9"
22	22.7	23.4	24.1	25	25.7	26.4	27.4	28.1	5'8"
22.8	23.5	24.2	24.9	25.9	26.6	27.3	28.4	29.1	5"7"
23.4	24.1	24.8	25.5	26.6	27.3	28	29	29.8	5'6"
24.2	25	25.7	26.4	27.5	28.3	29	30.1	30.8	5'5"
24.8	25.6	26.3	27.1	28.2	29	29.7	30.9	31.6	5'4"
25.8	26.6	27.3	28.1	29.3	30.1	30.9	32	32.8	5'3"
26.4	27.2	28	28.8	30	30.8	31.6	32.8		5'2"
27.5	28.3	29.1	30	31.2	32	32.9			5'1"
28.2	29	29.9	30.8	32	32.9				5'
29.3	30.2	31.1	32						4'11"
30.1	31	32	32.9						4'10"
66	68	70	72	75	77	79	82	84	

Height in feet and inches

Weight in kilograms

Index Chart

Waist to Hip Ratios

Hip measurement in cm

Waist (in) \ Hip cm	63	66	69	71	74	76	79	81	84	86	89	91	94	96	99	102	104	107	109	112	114	Waist cm
36	1.44	1.38	1.33	1.29	1.24	1.20	1.16	1.13	1.09	1.06	1.03	1.00	0.97	0.95	0.92	0.90	0.88	0.86	0.84	0.82	0.80	91
35	1.40	1.35	1.30	1.25	1.21	1.17	1.13	1.09	1.06	1.03	1.00	0.97	0.95	0.92	0.90	0.88	0.85	0.83	0.81	0.80	0.78	89
34	1.36	1.31	1.26	1.21	1.17	1.13	1.10	1.06	1.03	1.00	0.97	0.94	0.92	0.89	0.87	0.85	0.83	0.81	0.79	0.77	0.76	86
33	1.32	1.27	1.22	1.18	1.14	1.10	1.06	1.03	1.00	0.97	0.94	0.92	0.89	0.87	0.85	0.83	0.80	0.79	0.77	0.75	0.73	84
32	1.28	1.23	1.19	1.14	1.10	1.07	1.03	1.00	0.97	0.94	0.91	0.89	0.86	0.84	0.82	0.80	0.78	0.76	0.74	0.73	0.71	81
31	1.24	1.19	1.15	1.11	1.07	1.03	1.00	0.97	0.94	0.91	0.89	0.86	0.84	0.82	0.79	0.78	0.76	0.74	0.72	0.70	0.69	79
30	1.20	1.15	1.11	1.07	1.03	1.00	0.97	0.94	0.91	0.88	0.86	0.83	0.81	0.79	0.77	0.75	0.73	0.71	0.70	0.68	0.67	76
29	1.16	1.12	1.07	1.04	1.00	0.97	0.94	0.91	0.88	0.85	0.83	0.81	0.78	0.76	0.74	0.73	0.71	0.69	0.67	0.66	0.64	74
28	1.12	1.08	1.04	1.00	0.97	0.93	0.90	0.88	0.85	0.82	0.80	0.78	0.76	0.74	0.72	0.70	0.68	0.67	0.65	0.64	0.62	71
27	1.08	1.04	1.00	0.96	0.93	0.90	0.87	0.84	0.82	0.79	0.77	0.75	0.73	0.71	0.69	0.68	0.66	0.64	0.63	0.61	0.60	69
26	1.04	1.00	0.96	0.93	0.90	0.87	0.84	0.81	0.79	0.76	0.74	0.72	0.70	0.68	0.67	0.65	0.63	0.62	0.60	0.59	0.58	66
25	1.00	0.96	0.93	0.89	0.86	0.83	0.81	0.78	0.76	0.74	0.71	0.69	0.68	0.66	0.64	0.63	0.61	0.60	0.58	0.57	0.56	63
24	0.96	0.92	0.89	0.86	0.83	0.80	0.77	0.75	0.73	0.71	0.69	0.67	0.65	0.63	0.62	0.60	0.59	0.57	0.56	0.55	0.53	61
23	0.92	0.88	0.85	0.82	0.79	0.77	0.74	0.72	0.70	0.68	0.66	0.64	0.62	0.61	0.59	0.58	0.56	0.55	0.53	0.52	0.51	58
22	0.88	0.85	0.81	0.79	0.76	0.73	0.71	0.69	0.67	0.65	0.63	0.61	0.59	0.58	0.56	0.55	0.54	0.52	0.51	0.50	0.49	56
21	0.84	0.81	0.78	0.75	0.72	0.70	0.68	0.66	0.64	0.62	0.60	0.58	0.57	0.55	0.54	0.53	0.51	0.50	0.49	0.48	0.47	53
20	0.80	0.77	0.74	0.71	0.69	0.67	0.65	0.63	0.61	0.59	0.57	0.56	0.54	0.53	0.51	0.50	0.49	0.48	0.47	0.45	0.44	51
19	0.76	0.73	0.70	0.68	0.66	0.63	0.61	0.59	0.58	0.56	0.54	0.53	0.51	0.50	0.49	0.48	0.46	0.45	0.44	0.43	0.42	48
Waist (in) \ Hip in	25	26	27	28	29	30	31	32	33	34	35	36	37	38	39	40	41	42	43	44	45	

Hip measurement in inches

The Best Way to Lose Weight

Any idiot can write a book or magazine article which can help you lose weight. The problem is that none of these diets can **keep** the weight off. Think about it, if they really could, there would be no need to keep publishing new books and new articles, would there? If some of the most famous and wealthy people in the world, such as Oprah Winfrey, can't manage to keep weight off by using all of the 'top diets', doesn't this tell us two obvious things:

- Diets don't work.
- Whether they like it or not, these people were probably not meant to be particularly slim.

Never be taken in by diet claims of 'fast weight loss'. Speed is a **bad** thing when it comes to losing weight – you're more likely to put it straight back on, plus extra.

Everyone – whether they need to lose weight or not – will improve their health and body shape by remaining **physically active** and by having a **low-fat** diet. These are not temporary measures but a way of life which, unlike 'low-calorie diets', will enable you to achieve, and more importantly **maintain**, a healthy and more attractive body weight and shape. This may seem too simple to be true but it is the **only effective approach**. People who write 'diet' books and sell 'diet' products would like you to think otherwise!

To begin to put this into practice, read Chapters 4 and 9.

If you are below your healthy BMI and have a low WHR because you are constantly worried about being fat and you've been trying to slim, then please read Chapter 5.

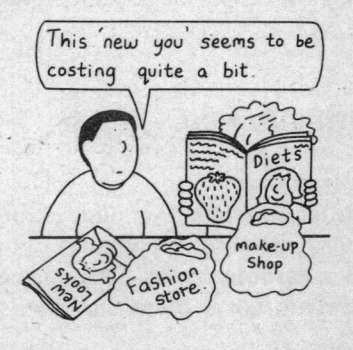

Chapter 4
Food

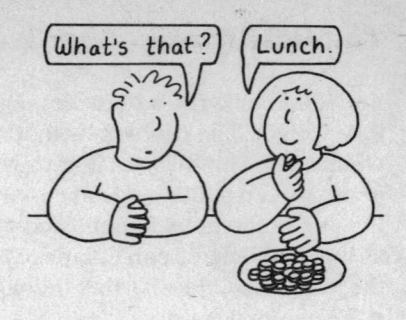

There was a scandal recently when scientists decided to look at exactly how low in fat the so-called 'low-fat' products on supermarket shelves actually were. They discovered that nearly half of them were actually very high in fat!

Most of the information we get about nutrition comes from those who sell us the food. Remember, they have a business to run and their claims are designed to make them a healthy profit. Whether you are healthy or not is *your* concern – not theirs. If you are interested in lowering your body mass index or simply want to know more about sound nutrition or a vegetarian diet, you can't rely upon adverts, manufacturers' claims or hearsay.

If you want detailed information on nutrition, it is available from the Health Education Authority or from school. I've chosen to discuss several food issues which are more relevant to you. It is essential, however, to understand first a few basic principles so you can make decisions about what you eat, based on fact – not fad.

Basic Elements of Food

Complex Carbohydrates
Otherwise known as starches, complex carbohydrates are the main source of *energy* in our diet, and most of our calories should come from complex carbohydrates. Examples are: potatoes, rice, porridge, pasta, bread, corn, plain shredded wheat or puffed

wheat, chappatis, sweet potatoes, green bananas, plaintains. They are **not** fattening and can help you lose weight and stay that way. It is best to eat wholegrain varieties – wholemeal bread or pasta, brown rice – because they contain more fibre, vitamins and minerals and are also more filling.

Protein
Protein is the basic material of life, needed for *growth* and *repair* of body tissues. Getting enough protein is not a problem for most young people in Britain. Many people wrongly believe that the more protein they get, the better. In fact, extra protein can also be burned for energy or changed into body fat and stored.

Vitamins and Minerals
These substances do not contain calories. They are substances which are necessary in tiny amounts for your body to function efficiently. You should easily be able to get all you need from a well-balanced diet and especially from fresh fruit and vegetables.

Fat and Low-Fat Eating

Fat comes in solid or liquid (oil) forms and while it is absolutely necessary to have some fat in our diets, most people still eat **too much fat**. While carbohydrates are the body's main source of energy, fats are the most concentrated source, and so high-fat foods are always high-calorie foods.

Fats are easily turned into body fat, the *storage material* for the body's extra energy supplies. Women have more body fat because back in prehistoric times when food was scarce, they had to have enough extra energy stored away to feed both themselves and breastfeed their babies. Men, on the other hand, had more muscle and less fat because they couldn't have babies or breastfeed and would instead have to search and hunt for food, so they simply needed lean power. While all of this may seem unnecessary and out of date now, our bodies and hormones don't change merely to suit the high-tech lives we lead today. This is precisely why diets don't work. Your body is still back in prehistoric times and when you suddenly reduce your food intake, it reacts as if it were still threatened with starvation by slowing down the rate at which it burns up calories, and by storing as much spare fat as possible – a survival mechanism. We cannot shake off our past just because it seems inconvenient. If it wasn't for our ability to store extra energy for future use, the human race wouldn't be here today. The problem is that nowadays, we eat when we like and no longer need to store our energy supplies for a rainy day the way we used to.

There are two well-known types of fat: *saturated fat* (or *saturates*) usually *raise* the cholesterol level in your blood which clogs arteries causing heart disease and strokes. The main sources of saturated fats are animal sources including butter, milk fat, cream, ghee and the fat in all meats; tropical oils such as coconut or palm also have lots of saturates.

Unsaturated fat (or *unsaturates*) tend to *lower* the cholesterol level in your blood. *Monounsaturates* are most easily found in olive oil. *Polyunsaturates* are found in corn, sunflower, sesame, soya and rapeseed oils. Oily fish such as mackerel, herring, sardines and pilchards contain a particularly useful form of polyunsaturates.

The Fat Con

A manufacturing process called *hydrogenation* makes unsaturated fat more saturated. Many foods now contain *hydrogenated vegetable oil* or fat because it makes them more firm and thick (like lard). Depending on the degree of hydrogenation, these artificially saturated vegetable fats are just as bad as the saturated fats we mentioned above. Read the ingredients list, as manufacturers slip them into a wide variety of foods.

When it comes to making you fat – fat is fat. No matter what type of fat you eat, if you eat too much they are all equally as good at making you fatter. The key is to keep the amount of *overall* fat you eat to an acceptable level and take in only a small amount of saturates compared to unsaturates.

Reducing Your Body Fat

Calories (actually called *kilocalories* and displayed as *kcal*) mean the amount of energy released when food is digested. It is the butter or margarine (fats) **not** the bread (carbohydrate) that can make you fat. Each gram of fat contains 9 calories, whereas the same weight of carbohydrate or protein contains only 4 calories, and this is why fat is more 'fattening' than carbohydrate or protein. In addition to this, some scientists now believe that the body may be able to turn dietary fat into body fat more easily than it can turn carbohydrate into body fat. In other words all calories are not equal – 100 calories of butter are more fattening than 100 calories of bread. This is why diets based on you counting your calories are a **waste of time**.

Quite simply, the most efficient way to reduce your body fat is to cut down on high-fat foods and eat a greater proportion of foods which are bulky and filling but lower in calories (such as carbohydrates, fruits and vegetables), and to stay physically active. It is worth repeating that carbohydrates, particularly the wholegrain variety, are **not** fattening. They only become fattening if they are cooked or served with fat. For example, while a 75-gram serving of boiled, microwaved or baked potatoes is worth about 140 calories, the same weight of chips contains **three times** as

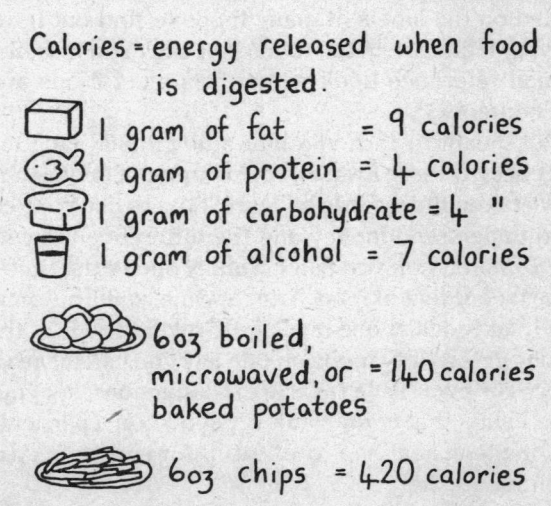

Calories = energy released when food is digested.

- 1 gram of fat = 9 calories
- 1 gram of protein = 4 calories
- 1 gram of carbohydrate = 4 "
- 1 gram of alcohol = 7 calories

- 6oz boiled, microwaved, or baked potatoes = 140 calories
- 6oz chips = 420 calories

many calories – and remember, those extra calories are **fat** calories, which may be easier to store as body fat than simply eating three times as many plain potatoes! Just for your information, alcohol is nice and fattening at 7 calories a gram, and so if you want to put on some extra blubber, drinking is a great way to do it (see 'Alcohol' in Chapter 7) and just think – you can kill your own brain cells at the same time as growing a pot belly!

You must never try to cut out all fat from your diet. Some scientists even believe that this could actually reduce the ability of your brain cells to absorb *serotonin*, a chemical that affects your mood, and that this could lead to extreme depression with its potentially dangerous consequences.

How to Reduce Dietary Fat

Everybody – whether they want to lose weight or not – should get **no more** than 30 per cent of their daily calories from fat. Some health professionals say the figure should be 20 per cent; most of you probably get 40 per cent. There's little point in giving you a mathematical formula for calculating exactly how many grams of fat you are 'allowed' every day – that would just complicate matters. You must, however, make use of the nutritional information provided on the labels of many foods to find out how much and what type of fats are in the foods you eat. (You may also wish to get a small reference book which lists most foods and their nutritional contents.)

This is not meant to turn you into a nutritional fanatic but to make you generally more aware of the amount of fat you currently eat. If you've taken the trouble to 'learn' how to use your cassette player or to understand money and the difference between a 5p coin and a £5 note, then you can certainly spend the time understanding the fat content of food. After a while, you'll automatically *balance* high-fat foods at one meal with low-fat foods at the next, or if you 'splurge' on fatty foods on one day you can make up for it the day after (or exercise a bit more). Remember, it's your **long term** eating habits that count – not a 'pig-out' on a particular day. This is a permanent, healthy way of eating for everyone – a diet for life **not** a slimming diet.

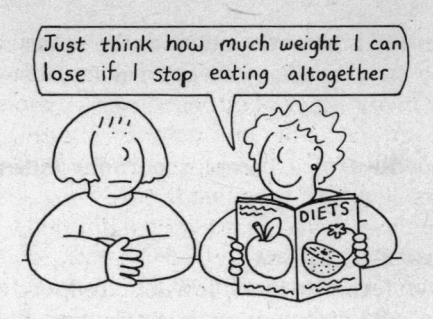

Tips on Reducing Dietary Fat

So, you need to cut down the amount of fat in your diet and make sure that most of it is unsaturated. Here are a few simple tips on how you can go about it.

• Use skimmed or semi-skimmed milk and low-fat milk products (such as yoghurt and cottage cheese), instead of full-fat types.

• Use less fats and oils. If you use margarine, choose one that has at least twice as much polyunsaturated fats as saturated fats. The best are only available from health food stores; they are not hydrogenated to make them firm.

• Bake, boil, steam, poach, grill or microwave foods instead of frying them in fat. If you do fry, use a non-stick pan with no oil.

• Butter and margarine are equally fattening so if you use them spread them more thinly. Don't use them in sandwiches just for the sake of it. British people have a terrible habit of using mayonnaise and butter together in a sandwich, and butter or margarine with beans on toast or grilled cheese sandwich!

• Make salad dressing with less oil or use low-fat yoghurt and loads of herbs, vinegar, tomato juice and spices instead of salad cream.

• Substitute low-fat fillings or ingredients for high-fat ones. Baked potatoes with beans, cottage cheese, tuna fish and no butter or margarine; low-fat yoghurt or low-fat fromage frais for cream; sorbet for ice cream.

- Most cheeses are high in fat, but with the range of cheese now available in the supermarket you can select those that are less high in fat.

- Increase your intake of complex carbohydrates, fresh vegetables and fruits.

Beware of 'Low-Fat' Claims

Many foods have terms such as 'low fat', 'reduced fat', 'light', or 'light in calories', which appear on the packaging. These terms are purely advertising claims **not** accurate nutritional information – in other words they're meaningless. Read the nutritional information label instead. While, for instance, a so-called 'low-fat' margarine or spread is lower in fat than regular butter or margarine, it still contains about 40 per cent fat.

Snacks and Junk Food

While most people should know that biscuits, sticky buns, cakes and ice cream are full of fat, there are plenty of other fatty snacks you may be less aware of. For example, about 65 per cent of the calories in crisps come from fat, even 'low-fat' crisps are 50 per cent fat calories. A bag of peanuts contain 75 per cent fat calories, 'Hoops' contain 56 per cent fat calories, and samosas are just dripping with fat calories. Most 'fast food' or take-aways are full of fat. Many of the snacks above are also very high in salt, which can lead to high blood pressure and to further health problems such as heart and kidney disease. Finally, chocolate tastes wonderful but it is basically just fat and sugar. The point is, to think about *how much* junk food you eat and to *cut down* on it – if you eat a lot, cut down on it drastically. By the way, don't automatically trust 'healthy' candy bars such as muesli and raisin – read the ingredients.

Example of Nutritional Information Food Label

kJ is short for kilojoules – an alternative way of measuring energy value.

The number of calories there are in 100 grams of this food.

NUTRITION INFORMATION	
100g provides	
Energy	1475kJ/346kcal
Protein	10.5 g
Carbohydrate	80g
(of which sugars)	2g
Fat	0.5g
(of which polyunsaturates	0.4g
and saturates)	0.1g
Sodium	0.3g
Fibre	6.2g

'Carbohydrate' is a blanket term which includes all sugars as well as wholesome complex carbohydrates.

Sometimes manufacturers are honest enough to tell you how much of the carbohydrate is actually sugar.

How much salt (sodium) there is in 100 grams of this food. We generally eat about 20 times more salt than we need.

How much saturated fat there is in 100 grams of this food. Choose foods with the lowest amount.

Vegetarian Eating

There are a variety of vegetarian diets ranging from 'vegan', which is strictly vegetarian and avoids all foods associated with animals including dairy products and eggs, to semi-vegetarian, which allows fish occasionally. Most people who describe themselves as vegetarians are 'lacto-ovovegetarian' meaning they don't eat meat or fish but do eat dairy products and eggs. Studies show that vegetarians may be less at risk from heart disease, diabetes and certain cancers and tend to have lower blood pressure, cholesterol levels, and weight. Studies also show that they generally live healthier life styles, exercising more and smoking and drinking less.

However, it is important to realise that a vegetarian diet can also be very unhealthy if you make poor food choices. For example, cheeses, full-fat milk, cream, ice cream, butter, oils, peanut butter, cakes, sweets, crisps, white bread, soft drinks and alcohol can also constitute a complete vegetarian diet but would be high in fat, salt, sugar and alcohol, and low in fibre. It is therefore just as important to consider the general principles of nutrition whether you are a vegetarian or not. These are outlined at the end of this chapter. Lacto-ovo and semi-vegetarians generally choose from all the basic food groups and should be no more likely to suffer from a lack of nutrients than a meat eater. Vegans, on the other hand, must ensure that they plan their diets a bit more carefully or they could wind up with certain deficiencies such as vitamins B12 and D; the minerals calcium, iron and zinc; and protein. If you are vegan or are thinking of becoming vegan, don't simply cut out all meat, fish, dairy products and eggs without understanding the principles of a good vegan diet. It's worth contacting The Vegetarian Society for helpful information. Send a stamped addressed envelope to:

The Vegetarian Society UK Ltd, Parkdale, Dunham Road, Altringham WA14 4QG

It is important to eat a wide variety of foods: fruits, vegetables, complex carbohydrates (especially the wholegrain variety), legumes (such as beans, nuts, chick-peas, butter beans, lentils, seeds and soya products) and if possible include low-fat dairy products and eggs occasionally, to get a full range of nutrients.

While many legumes and grains are good sources of protein, they have to be combined to make them usable for the body. For example, combine legumes with wholegrain bread, rice or cereal. Many people wrongly believe that you have to combine these complimentary foods in the same meal to get the effects of a 'complete' protein. If you eat the complimentary foods within a few hours of one another, that will do the trick.

'Problem' Parents!

Some parents are becoming increasingly aware of the dietary issues we have been talking about and are working to improve the diets of themselves and their families. But not all of them!

Your parents may be a problem. They come from a generation which has some of the worst eating habits in the world. If they do the shopping or cooking, your diet is very much at their mercy. It's a good idea to educate them about nutrition, possibly showing them this chapter. It's *not* a good idea to start the conversation with phrases like, 'Mummy, why are you killing me with blubber foods – I thought you loved me'. After all, how would **you** react to that kind of approach! Leaving 'healthy eating' booklets from the Health Education Authority around the house may help, but you must talk to them – they may be in blissful ignorance of the real facts. And how about helping with the shopping and cooking so that you can buy what you want and prepare foods in a healthier way? There's nothing like taking the solution into your own hands.

Facts and Myths about Diet

We have already explained the basis of a good diet. Here is the truth about a few more topics you may have heard discussed.

Breakfast and Your 'Weight'
Studies show that breakfast speeds up your metabolism which burns calories and helps keep you feeling more energetic for the rest of the day. You will also be less likely to binge on high-fat, high-calorie foods later on. Skipping breakfast slows your

metabolism down by 3 to 4 per cent which can make you feel sluggish, even a bit depressed. So any of you who may consider skipping breakfast should realize that a slower metabolism and the additional snacking can actually add 3 to 4 kilograms of pure blubber to your body each year. Don't skip the most important meal of the day.

Television Makes You Fat
While TV 'rays' don't force fat on to your bones, watching lots of telly **has** been linked to obesity. People who watch three hours or more a day are twice as likely to be obese as those who watch less than an hour. This is because it prevents you from being active so you don't burn up calories, you put on extra fat. This becomes a cycle, because if you are unfit and have too much body fat, you would rather sit in front of a telly, as it becomes too much effort to get up and do anything. Adverts also encourage you to eat more high-calorie snacks. One scientist has evidence that watching television slows down the rate at which you burn calories, compared to reading or even 'doing nothing'.

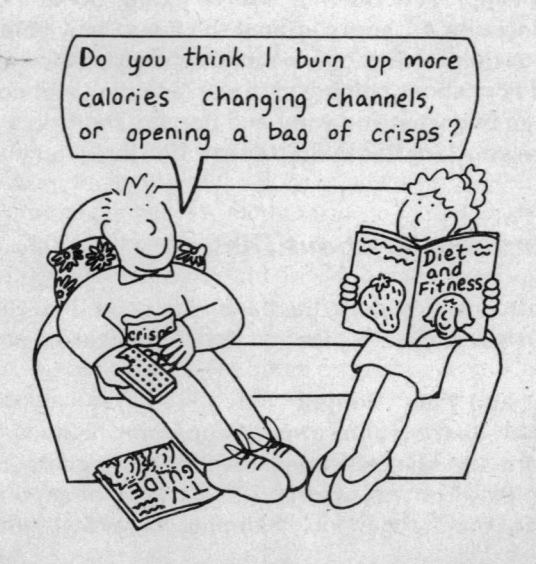

High-Protein Diets and Muscles

Many people try to eat more protein to improve athletic performance, to have a stronger body or bigger muscles or even to improve the condition of their hair or nails. High-protein diets are completely useless and so are the high-tech, high-protein powders, liquids, tablets, bars etc. The only way to build muscle is to exercise, and you should eat the same healthy diet we discussed above. High-protein diets can also put a strain on the kidneys.

Are Vitamin Tablets Useful?

For most people the answer is **no**. Taking extra vitamins or minerals will not give you better-looking skin or hair, make you live longer, or make you a better athlete – despite what you hear. Many people stupidly believe that 'if a little is necessary, a lot is better' and take large doses of particular vitamins or minerals. This is not only useless but can actually be toxic, damaging your liver and nerve cells. Taking extra vitamin C, for example, will **not** prevent colds but it can give you stomach aches, diarrhoea or kidney stones.

Apart from this, vitamin tablets don't work as well as obtaining vitamins in your food. In fact, many don't work at all, passing straight through your body – money literally down the drain. Anyone with a reasonably well-balanced diet won't gain a thing from vitamin tablets. You cannot make up for a poor diet by taking tablets – **it doesn't work!**

Sugar, Glucose and 'Quick Energy'

Glucose, dextrose, sugar or any sweets **do not** provide quick energy, although many sports drinks and sweet manufacturers, as well as the sugar industry, would like you to think they do. White table sugar (*sucrose*) is only one form of sugar. Some other names for sugar are *barley malt, dextrose, fructose, glucose, honey, invert syrup, lactose, maltose, mannitol molasses, sorbitol*. All sugars are pretty much the same and none has any significant advantage over the other, although molasses does contain iron. There is no difference between white sugar, brown sugar and honey. The sugar in fruits such as peaches, oranges and melons is the same type of sugar as that found in a chocolate bar. The difference is that the refined table sugar is empty calories – it has no nutritional value whatsoever – and, what's more, it rots your teeth! The fruit, on the other hand, contains other valuable nutritional elements, such as vitamins and fibre.

Your body makes its own glucose from the complex carbohydrates you eat and even from protein and fat. Eating or drinking glucose (also called dextrose) products is unnecessary and can actually make you less energetic. So if you want to win a match you'd really be better off offering any sweet things, glucose or dextrose products to the other team. While having low blood sugar levels can make you feel tired and sluggish, taking any form of sugar will actually make your blood sugar drop even lower than before. This may seem the opposite of what you would expect, but this is how it happens. When you consume sugar, your pancreas releases lots of insulin to deal with the sugar by helping cells to absorb it and use it as energy, or by storing it in your liver or muscles to be used as energy later. However, because we weren't designed to deal with large amounts of pure sugar, the pancreas may over-react and produce too much insulin, which removes too much of the sugar from your bloodstream leaving you with less than you started with. On the other hand, many complex carbohydrates cause less of a 'glucose rebound' effect. Our bodies weren't built to handle sugars, they need to make their own – don't let anyone tell you differently. (See 'Sports Drinks' in Chapter 9.) By the way, don't trust labels like 'no added sugar' or 'sugar-free', check the ingredients yourself for the other names for sugar. Bread, for example, often has glucose syrup, invert syrup or dextrose listed – but no mention of sugar! How sweet of them to fool us.

Calcium Alert
New studies suggest that pre-teens, who get three times the recommended daily requirement of calcium (500 mg), grow stronger, denser bones. This is the most critical period for bone development and may also help prevent many fractures and the likelihood of osteoporosis (when bones become thin, brittle and fragile in 60–70-year-olds – usually women). The message is that girls in particular must ensure they get more calcium, both before and during puberty (ages 9–14). Of course, you should try to maintain this afterwards as well. Aim to get around 1200–1500 mg

of calcium per day from the food you eat – tablets or supplements are not good substitutes for low-fat yoghurt or low-fat milk, broccoli, greens, spinach etc. Boys should also take note – these are your foundation years when you are building your body's framework – so make the most of them.

Anti-Cancer Diets

As many as a third of all cancers are linked to diet, high-fat diets in particular. There are also other foods that may increase our risk of cancers. If you follow a sensible balanced diet and are aware of particular areas to avoid, you automatically reduce the health risks. You don't need to avoid these foods altogether, just don't have them too regularly.

- When vegetable oil is heated to fry foods, it breaks down and can produce *free radicals* – unstable molecules that may damage body cells and cause cancer. Frying also increases the fat in your diet, which is again linked to cancers.

- Cured, smoked and pickled foods such as hot dogs, ham and various pickled cucumbers are high in *nitrites* and *nitrates*, which in high amounts are linked to cancers.

- When your body burns alcohol it produces *acetaldehyde* which is a potential cancer-causing substance. Drinking also increases the effectiveness of the other cancer-causing substances in foods and tobacco. (See 'Alcohol' in Chapter 7.)

On the other side of the scale, scientists now believe that eating several helpings of certain fruits and vegetables each day, will provide us with substances such as *sulforaphane*, *indoles* and *betacarotene* which may help prevent certain cancers. The good guys are:

- Cruciferous vegetables such as broccoli, cauliflower, Brussels sprouts, cabbage (microwaved or steamed preferably).

- Fresh greens, yellows and reds – raw is best – such as spinach and peppers.

- Fruits and vegetables containing vitamins A and C – such as beans, carrots, lettuce, tomatoes and apricots – these will also help to prevent heart attacks.

Putting it all together

Despite all the information that we are bombarded with, the principles of a healthy diet are really very simple:

1 Eat a diet high in complex carbohydrates.
2 Eat at least five servings of fruits and vegetables per day, especially cruciferous vegetables, fresh greens, and yellow and red fruits and vegetables, and those high in vitamins A and C.
3 No more than 30 per cent of your calories should come from fat – preferably less. Make sure that you avoid too much saturated fat or hydrogenated oils.
4 Make sure you get at least 1200 milligrams of calcium a day from low-fat foods such as low-fat milk, yoghurt and green vegetables.
5 Limit the amount of salt (sodium) you take in by not adding it to your food, asking your parents not to add it to cooking (they can add their own afterwards), avoiding salty foods and reading food labels as most sodium comes from processed foods. We already consume about twenty times more salt than we need.
6 Avoid sugar. In addition to rotting your teeth, many foods that are high in sugar are also high in fat. Sugar is 'empty' calories.
7 Eat a variety of foods. This will ensure that you get all the nutrients you need and will also limit your exposure to any pesticides or toxins that may be found in one particular food.
8 If you haven't started drinking alcohol, don't bother taking up the habit. Don't be conned into believing that 'moderate' or 'sensible' drinking is actually better for you than not drinking at all.
9 Make use of the nutritional information and ingredients listed on food labels.

Remember – educate your parents about these issues. *Bon appetit* and good luck!

Chapter 5
Fear of Food

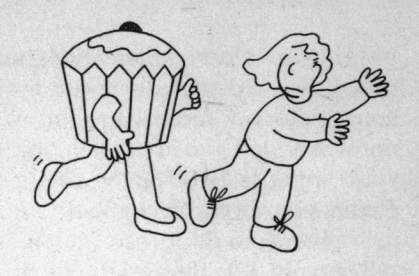

There is a very telling scene in a movie called *Eating*. A number of women are sitting around a table celebrating a birthday, the candles are blown out on the birthday cake and the first piece is cut and passed around and passed around and around and around – every woman trying to avoid 'the chocolate enemy'.

It is generally true to say that while boys simply eat food, girls have a *relationship* with food. Many of you feel guilty if you feel you've eaten too much. Food can be seen as more than merely nutritious or not nutritious, tasting good or not tasting so good – it becomes an issue that you have to cope with – it is even considered by some as the enemy which must be battled against. At the same time, being overweight is thought of as bad and disgusting, while being thin is good and beautiful.

Food has always been a symbol of love and survival. After all, the first thing a baby does when it's born (apart from crying, that is) is to breastfeed. Feeding not only helps mother and baby to bond but also helps families and friends to become, or remain, closer by participating in a common activity together – eating. However, for someone who suffers a loss or is emotionally hurt or upset, food may take on a strangely different meaning. Their appetite becomes their 'voice' to cry out with as they search for a way to say things about themselves – based upon food and styles of eating. Food is something which must somehow be *controlled*.

It is important to mention that many people find that their appetite is affected by their emotions. For example, depression may cause you to lose your appetite temporarily or stress may lower your blood sugar levels and make you eat more sugary things. Some distressing event may trigger such an effect on your appetite for a few days on a one-off basis, in which case you must not worry that you are developing an eating disorder. However, if your appetite is strongly affected by something that has happened, you should recognize it and get it off your chest by talking to someone about it (see Chapter 6).

There is a wide variety of problems with eating related to unhappiness and illness. The two most well-known problems are *anorexia nervosa* and *bulimia nervosa*. You may recognize some of the characteristics of people who have these problems – either in yourself or someone close to you. The study of eating disorders is not an exact science and so you may find that your behaviour doesn't fit neatly into either category. However, many of the basic feelings involved also apply to other eating disorders, such as *compulsive* eating and *over-eating*.

The first thing to realize is that eating disorders are **not** really about food. They are about deep-seated emotional conflict and unhappiness. Food and eating are used as a language to express difficulties and unhappiness. Eating disorders are:

- A way of *avoiding* issues. By focusing all her attention on food and eating, a person can avoid facing more painful things in her life.

- A way of *coping* when someone's life seems to be full of problems with no solutions.

- A way of feeling in *control* of one's own body and life in general when someone may feel that other people or events are trying to control them.

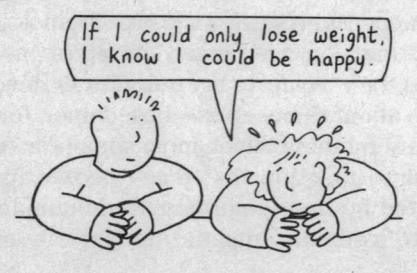

- A way of reacting to the stress someone may be experiencing now or due to an event in the past.

People with eating disorders have a few things in common. They are overcome by the attitude our society has – that the way you look is more important than it ever was and certainly more important than your 'inner' qualities. They are terrified of becoming fat and are driven to become slim. They are obsessed with food, calories, weight and body shape. They rely on eating, and/or avoiding eating, as a way of coping. Deep inside they often feel worthless and have a very low opinion of themselves. They usually find it very difficult, even frightening, to accept that they have an eating disorder and will deny this problem even when others draw their attention to it.

It isn't clear yet whether anorexia and bulimia are completely separate problems or different versions of the same problem. Some people who are anorexic also do some of the things that bulimics do, and many bulimics used to be anorexic.

What Causes Eating Disorders?

People like to look for a single cause of an eating disorder. For example, anorexia is often described as a 'slimmer's disease'. However, eating disorders are probably the result of a number of things which a person experiences. Here are some examples, but please remember that different people are affected by a different combination of things in a slightly different way. There are plenty of other possible causes, but these are enough to be going on with for now.

Family
Many people feel that their family's expectations of them are too high and that they have to *achieve* and *accomplish* things in order to feel *valued* and important within their family. Even if they are mistaken in believing this, the effect is the same, for they set high goals for themselves which they cannot reach. This leaves them feeling dissatisfied with themselves. In order to cope with these painful feelings they turn to something which they feel they can control – food and weight.

Mothers can have a very powerful effect on their daughters, who may feel that they are being *controlled* by Mum. Mothers may also not help their daughters to feel attractive and may actually *criticize* the way they look. Mothers have a special invisible way of approving or disapproving of you or what you do that's very hard to put your finger on, but nevertheless very effective. Fathers may make a comment about you having a 'big bottom' quite innocently, but you may take this to heart and be hurt or worried about it.

Refusing to eat may seem the only way to show your feelings or send a message to your family. This often results in a struggle between you and your parents – a battle for control.

Dieting
Dieting may seem the solution to your emotional problems because it allows you to take control of something. But like drugs, the solution takes control of you and itself becomes the problem.

Emotional Problems
Being upset about a death, trouble with friends, your parents' divorce or simply a big change in your life like going to a new school, even if it isn't a bad experience, can trigger eating problems.

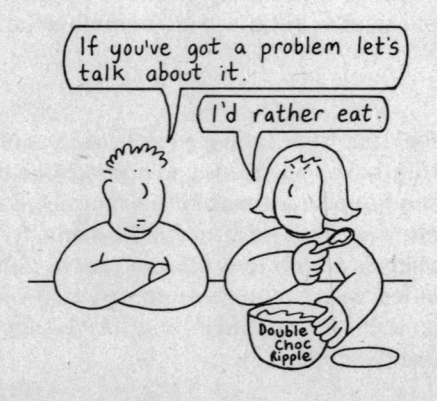

Adolescence
Turning from a girl into a woman involves your body, as well as your feelings, going through big changes. By slowing down or stopping your body from changing into a grown woman, anorexia can seem to be a way of regaining control of your changing body, thereby avoiding all the demands of growing up.

The Pressure to be 'Slim'
We discussed this in Chapter 3. Our culture believes you can never be too rich or too slim. As a result, almost everyone tries to diet at some point – some get drawn in over their heads. In cultures where there is no pressure to be thin, eating disorders are extremely rare.

Inheritance
Inheriting your parents' ability to develop an eating disorder through genes or picking up your mother's own concern about her weight are both thought to be possible.

Sexual Abuse
Sexual abuse can often make girls feel bad – even guilty about their bodies and this can lead to bad feelings towards their bodies and a lack of self-esteem.

Anorexia Nervosa

Anorexia usually starts with a diet to lose weight, but once you lose weight you're not satisfied and want to continue slimming. No matter who says 'you're too thin', you don't believe them and feel strongly that you're still overweight and must lose more. While other people may think you've simply lost your appetite, you are in fact extremely interested in food but terrified of being fat. You may disguise the fact that you're dieting by eating large amounts of 'light' foods – fruit, vegetables and salads which have hardly any calories – and avoiding essential calories from carbohydrates, for example, so you dwindle away. You may also do a lot of vigorous exercise.

68   FEAR OF FOOD

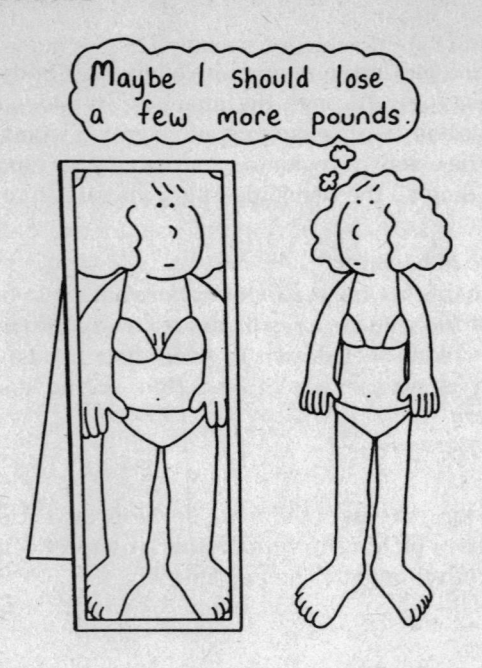

Maybe I should lose a few more pounds.

By this stage, your body mass index has dropped to below 21, although you probably think that the body mass index or the usual height/weight charts are too 'generous' and are not a good way for you to judge whether you are a good weight or not. If you normally have monthly periods, they have probably stopped. The thought of being with other people when you might be expected to eat lots of food with them, scares you. You also become more of a loner and more secretive because of the kind of life you lead and the way you feel about yourself. You may become hyperactive and restless and even find it difficult to sleep properly. The amount of weight you've lost has upset your hormones, which has not only upset your menstrual cycle but can cause you to grow downy hair on your body and you may even lose some hair from your head. As your body has no fuel, you may feel cold and have poor circulation in your hands and feet.

If after reading this far, you recognize yourself in any of the descriptions, then you must **start to help yourself**. Your life **can** actually be much happier, even though this may seem an impossibility right now. Information on how to do this is available a few pages on from here. Even if your body mass index hasn't actually dropped below 21 (girls) or 22 (boys) yet, it is absolutely necessary to deal with this problem as soon as possible as it can easily get out of hand, and the sooner you start to help yourself, the sooner you will feel happier. You probably wouldn't have read this far in the first place if the whole issue of food wasn't a problem for you, or someone you know. You can still be an anorexic in thought without actually losing weight. In other words, if you're starting to have these feelings now, you could be on the road to more serious problems if you don't act.

Anorexic Feelings

The way you see yourself and your problems is what is *really* making you over concerned with food, calories, weight and body shape. In many ways, you may see yourself as a failure, no matter how much success you have in other people's eyes. You feel that others are better looking, slimmer, brighter, more talented. You also believe that other people see you this way – even your family and friends. You feel inadequate – no matter what you do, it will not be good enough. Some people would see you as a perfectionist with unrealistically high standards. The fact that you are in some way unhappy, confused, under stress, makes you reach for some *control* and the one thing that you feel sure will give you a sense of achievement is the act of controlling your **weight**. After all, it's a simple 'religion' really: *good* and *evil*, *success* and *failure*, can be neatly measured by numbers on a scale or calories in food. By concentrating on this you can avoid the unhappiness involved in concentrating on you, your feelings, your relationships with others and accepting your own strengths and limitations.

The problem with this way of coping is that it is a two-edged sword. You may feel a sense of achievement when you lose weight but you will feel crushed, defeated and even more of a failure if you gain weight. That 'control lever' is always slightly out of reach . . . 'if only I weighed a few kilos less, life would be so much better'. In reality, you have **lost** control because your concern about food, calories and weight is actually controlling **you**.

Boys and Anorexia

Although girls who are anorexic outnumber boys by about fifteen to one, an increasing number of boys are being found who also have anorexic behaviour. In fact, even some famous men are now thought to have been anorexic. Lewis Carroll, author of *Alice in Wonderland* and Oxford lecturer, never went in for dinner, but spent his time collecting and reading the dinner menus instead. Another famous novelist, Franz Kafka, worked as a manager in an insurance company and used to leave the sandwiches his mother made him for the cleaning lady. This wasn't because he was a nice guy, nor because his mother made lousy sandwiches, it now appears that he was simply anorexic.

Nowadays boys can more easily disguise anorexic behaviour through more acceptable means, such as tremendous amounts of physical exercise. Many of these boys place a lot of importance on being *successful* and *achieving* things. An additional problem that boys have is that they may be less willing to seek help, and at the same time many people normally expect girls to be the ones who seem anorexic.

Bulimia Nervosa

Bulimic behaviour involves binge-eating or 'pigging out' on enormous quantities of high-calorie foods – and then trying to clean it all out by making yourself vomit, starving yourself, or using laxative or diuretic medicines. Unlike anorexic behaviour, bulimics can usually manage to keep their weight within a normal range.

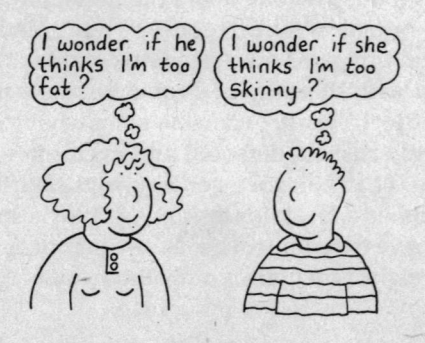

This is because when they binge, they often go for large amounts of particularly fattening foods such as chocolates, cakes, biscuits, butter and cheese, and their body manages to absorb some of it. While bulimia is predominantly a female problem, men in certain jobs such as modelling, jockeys and even male wrestlers appear to be more likely to suffer from bulimia.

Bulimic Feelings
Like anorexic feelings, bulimic feelings involve a very low sense of your own worth. However, many people who are bulimic often seem very confident, happy and successful from the outside – even though they are terribly miserable and depressed on the inside. Unlike anorexic behaviour which other people can see by the amount of weight you lose, bulimic behaviour can usually be kept secret. Bulimia creates even more guilt, shame, disgust and self-hatred than anorexia. While someone may appear to eat in front of others quite normally, they often go straight into the loo afterwards to get rid of the food they ate. This leaves them feeling even worse about themselves. While you **can't** control your overpowering desire to eat, you **can** control whether the food stays in your body, and because you may fear that once you start to eat, you won't be able to stop, you give in to your appetite and then undo it. You go completely out of control when you binge and then quickly try to regain control by emptying yourself. You may have started this vicious cycle because you felt anorexic before – terrified of becoming fat – now you want to eat but still stay thin. Bulimia may wrongly seem the perfect solution to these two opposing desires.

What Harm Can Eating Disorders Cause?

Anorexia **is** starvation, even though you may call it 'dieting'. Here are some of the affects of such extreme low-calorie dieting.

- Depression. Even though you may be dieting *because* you are unhappy, the chemical effects in your brain caused by dieting are likely to make you even more unhappy.

- Difficulty in concentrating or thinking clearly. Your brain cells simply don't have enough nutrition to function normally.

- Brittle bones which start to dissolve and break easily.

- Broken sleep.

- The effects of extreme dieting make people so depressed that they attempt suicide or go past the point of no return and starve themselves to death. Others are so undernourished that they die from infections. This is not an exaggeration to scare you – please take it seriously.

- Vomiting causes the powerful *hydrochloric acid* from your stomach to burn away the enamel on your teeth. The salivary glands in your neck can become swollen, giving you a puffy face. Because you're losing important minerals, your heart may not be able to beat in a regular way – possibly leading to a heart attack. You could have epileptic-type fits, rupturing of your stomach, kidney damage and death.

- Laxatives can give you constant stomach pains, swollen fingers and long-term damage to your intestines with constipation.

- Diuretics work by making you urinate. These medicines cause dehydration and are very bad news.

Ask Yourself These Questions

Is your body mass index below 21 if you are a girl or 22 if you are a boy? (see pages 44–5)	Yes/No
If so, have you lost weight by controlling your eating?	Yes/No
Have your monthly periods stopped?	Yes/No
Has anyone told you that you look thin and should eat more?	Yes/No

Do you think about calories, food and avoiding food all the time?   Yes/No

Do you 'binge' – going totally out of control and eating enormous amounts of usually high-calorie foods – and then make yourself vomit, or starve yourself or use laxative or diuretic medicines?   Yes/No

Are you secretive about your eating–   Yes/No

If you have answered **yes** to any of these questions then you could have a problem – so please read on.

Help

There is no magic formula for 'curing' an eating disorder. As with many problems, the most important step is to recognize and accept that you have a problem. Learning more about the real reason for your problem with food and weight will enable you to come to terms with the true source – which is neither the food nor your weight. Although an eating disorder may end up as a 'medical' problem, it is almost always originally caused by troubled *emotions* and you can't avoid facing up to these without paying a terrible price. If you recognized yourself in this chapter then you already have an advantage.

Many people with an eating disorder are worried that if they ask for help, the medical authorities will be alerted and they will be examined by doctors in white coats and forced to eat. This is **not** the case! In fact the treatment for your eating disorder will be controlled by **you**.

There are now a number of ways that you can get help and information confidentially. For example, the **Eating Disorders Association** has a Youth Helpline which you can ring to discuss things with someone who will be sympathetic to your problem. You don't have to give your name and they can provide you with both understanding and support as well as information about local groups run by people who have the same eating problems that you do. You will not be judged or lectured at or told 'You're

74 FEAR OF FOOD

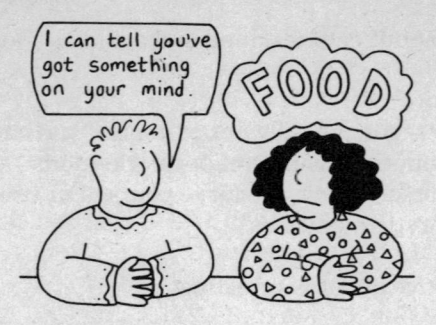

too thin – eat, eat'. Just talking to someone who has the same problem is **extremely helpful** and will be a relief. They can ring you back to save the cost of the call if you want. They will **never** tell anyone.

You will also be able to find out from them about all the methods of help available in your area. It is purely up to you if you want to look into these choices.

- Counselling is usually available. Talking privately with another person who is experienced in dealing with eating problems, and may well have had the same problems themselves, is extremely helpful.

- Family counselling involves some members of your family meeting with an experienced counsellor to discuss some of the family expectations and problems that contribute to eating problems.

- Group help means that people with the same eating problems meet to support one another or discuss issues.

- Sometimes a counsellor talks to a group of people, and sometimes their families as well, about eating problems.

- Nutritional counselling is available to help you deal with your fear of 'forbidden foods' and help you plan your own healthy meals so that you can eat without being terrified of getting fat.

A doctor can prescribe medication to help you if you are very depressed and suffering from an eating disorder. Here are some telephone numbers and addresses to help you or someone you know.

For anorexia and bulimia:
Eating Disorders Association, Sackville Place, 44 Magdalen Street, Norwich, Norfolk, NR3 1JU.
Youth Helpline 0603 765050 (4 p.m. to 6 p.m. Monday, Tuesday and Wednesday). They can ring you back to save you the cost of the call if you want.
Regular Helpline 0603 621414 (9 a.m. to 6.30 p.m. Monday to Friday) or 0490 521431 (11.30 a.m. to 2.30 p.m. Monday to Friday).

For over-eating or compulsive eating you can telephone **Overeaters Anonymous** which has a taped telephone message giving lists of self-help meetings and an address to write to. Their number is 071 275 8008.

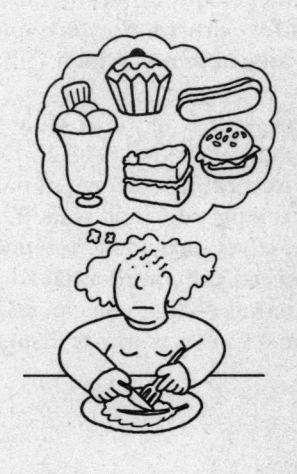

Chapter 6
Unhappiness

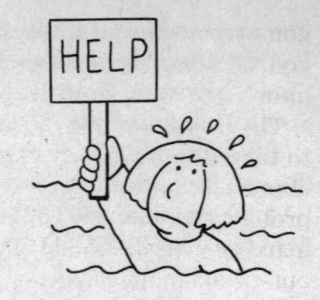

There is no shortage of things that can make you unhappy, and unhappiness comes in many different flavours. Some aspects overlap with, or lead to, others. For example, being bullied can make you anxious and nervous, which can make you sad and depressed.

Even though there seems to be a wide variety of different reasons for being unhappy, the solutions often come down to the same thing. Feeling miserable is a form of pain, and like any pain in your body, it is telling you that something needs attention. Wherever possible, I've provided telephone helplines and addresses where you can get confidential advice and information without giving your name, so that you can respond to your unhappiness and make some moves towards dispelling it.

Misery

Everyone feels depressed, sad and miserable at certain times in their life, and often with a specific reason – perhaps someone they were close to has died, for example. In many other cases, the person may not know exactly why they are unhappy. The point is, **you don't need a reason** for feeling miserable nor do you need a label for what you are feeling, whether it feels like deep sadness, depression, anger, stress, pressure, nervousness, fear, loneliness, confusion, guilt, shame or a combination of feelings. Feeling miserable is an important reaction to things in your *life* or things

UNHAPPINESS 77

going on in your *mind*. It tells you that something is not right for you, it spurs you to act and make decisions as you grow up based upon what feels good and bad for *you*.

The important thing is to recognize that you are not happy and to **take some action**. By doing something or talking to someone about the way you feel, you will definitely improve things. The problem often is that when you feel bad, you feel there is no point in trying to do anything; there is no answer, no choices and no way out – you actually lose your ability to see what really *can* be done to make you feel better. But something can always be done if you seek out the right help.

While it is abnormal not to have miserable times, what action you take is always a question of *how* miserable you actually are, *what* has made you feel this way (if you know), *how long* you've felt this and how it is affecting your everyday life.

Depression (feeling really, really low and sad or just cold, empty and numb) seems to be affecting more people at an earlier age than ever. Many of the reasons are to do with the way our society and our families have changed over the last twenty years, and the kinds of new pressures, expectations and disappointments that we feel at a younger and younger age. At the same time, our world seems less stable – global warming, AIDS, families splitting up, communities breaking down. We feel more *isolated* because there seem to be fewer people, things, systems and beliefs we can *rely* on – things change so quickly nowadays. When we do experience difficulties we need *stability* around us and *people* to rely on to help us get a grip on things. So let's look at where you can find that help and support, and why it is so important.

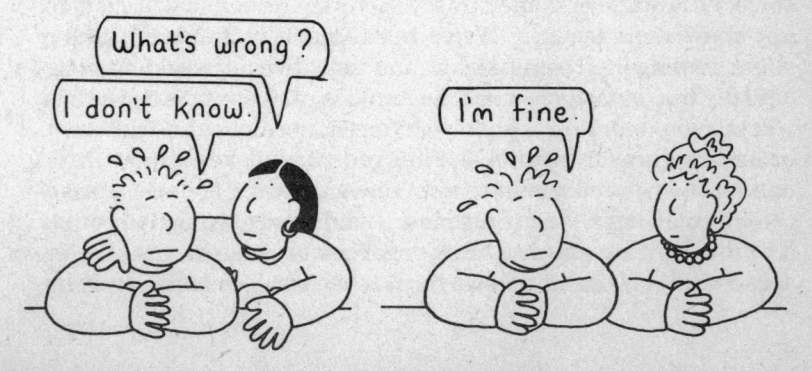

Letting Off Steam

After decades of experiments and billions of pounds worth of studies, science has discovered, not surprisingly, that *people need people*. Expressing your feelings to another understanding person is the best medicine science has found for making you happier. This may sound too simple and too obvious, but studies have even shown that by expressing emotions, you will actually improve your immune system and be less likely to catch disease! Even keeping a *written diary* of your inner feelings, thoughts and confessions which you may not dare to tell anybody, will improve your health, boost your immune system, and make you happier. You may not feel better immediately, but the emotional benefits will come in time, even if it takes several months.

The key to all of this is that, one way or the other, we must take time to explore our feelings and express our deepest beliefs. But life is too fast nowadays, there are too many choices and decisions to make, and we're too distracted by outside things to do – TV, video games, sports clubs – and so we miss out on taking time to look at our *inside* world.

This may sound wimpish and wet, almost like an American television show – especially, perhaps, to boys – but you cannot avoid this need or you'll pay a heavy price. Four out of five young people who kill themselves are boys. In addition to this, the numbers of young men who do commit suicide has increased by 75 per cent in the last ten years. Part of the reason for this is that boys generally find it much more difficult to talk about their feelings – and bottling up emotions *always* causes problems.

Boys shouldn't be blamed for this because even today our society's attitude is shaped by the Victorian principle that men do not show their feelings. We've been taught to think of talking about feelings as being sickly and sensitive – 'weak' – while actually the opposite is true. The families of many suicide victims will tell you that. Boys also have different hormones and different brain structures from girls and this probably makes it more difficult for them to talk about or even recognize their feelings. Unlike the caveman days, when only muscle and power seemed to count, it is now females who are the stronger sex because they are better able to fight off one of the real threats of today – unhappy feelings

– by simply talking about them, 'letting off steam' so the kettle doesn't explode.

While more boys succeed in committing suicide, the numbers of girls committing or attempting suicide has also increased. Many try to kill themselves, possibly hoping that someone will find them in time to save them and that people around them will realize how unhappy they are. Unfortunately, they are often wrong and are not rescued in time or they are left with damaged body organs such as their liver, or even with brain damage. Also people try to harm or injure themselves in various ways. While they are not actually attempting suicide, it is still a sign that they are seriously unhappy and need urgent help.

Who To Talk To
If you are very unhappy **for any reason** it always helps to talk to someone who will listen sympathetically. Having close friends is more important than getting the highest grades in school. It makes life a lot easier if you can talk to them when you're fed up or miserable. Brothers, sisters, parents, teachers, aunts, uncles, grandparents, GPs and even your vicar, can be very helpful in making you feel happier – **try talking** to some of them if you can.

If you feel there is no one close to you in whom you can confide, there are a number of phone numbers which you can ring any time, day or night, for confidential advice and help. You don't need to give your name. Remember you do not need to be 'suicidal' or have any particular problem that you can identify. If you are simply miserable or worried, or you want to help someone else who is, then please ring – they really do want to hear from you. You can ring the **Samaritans**, their number is inside the front cover of any local phone book or Directory Enquiries can give you the nearest number. The Samaritans can also arrange to meet with you, if you wish, or they can tell you who may specialize in helping you confidentially with your particular problem. You can also ring **Childline** free of charge on 0800 1111 or you can write to them free of charge at:

Freepost Childline, 1111 London N1 0BR.

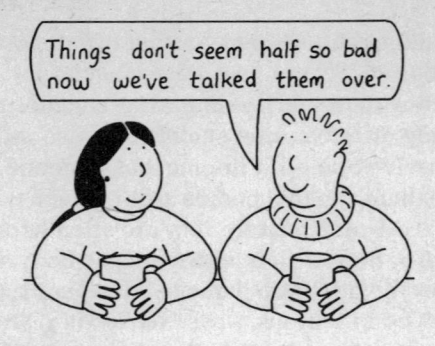

Writing Your Problems Down

Exploring your deepest thoughts and feelings on paper is not a cure for all problems, nor a substitute for getting help when you need it. But it can help you to cope with less severe unhappiness and it can also be used in addition to talking things out with others. What it will do is to give you a clearer understanding of what is going on and it will allow you to let off steam and look at worries more realistically. In many respects it's like exercise or a low-fat diet – as part of your lifestyle, it will help keep you healthy. You may also find that it helps you to sort out some answers to your problems.

What Should You Write About?
You don't need to write about the most upsetting thing that ever happened to you, but if you find yourself thinking about something too much of the time, writing about it can help you come to terms with it. Also, if there is something you feel you can't tell others about because you're embarrassed or scared of being punished, write about it.

How Should You Write?
Try to see your problems the way an outsider would and also include the way you actually feel about it. Just let go completely and say truthfully what you feel about it, and why you feel that way. Remember no one else will see this, so you may as well be honest with yourself. Keep writing and don't worry about spelling, grammar or presentation.

When and Where to Write

Try to write for about fifteen minutes a day in a place where you won't be disturbed or distracted by other things or people. The more special the setting, the better.

You might feel sad or depressed immediately afterwards or feel a great relief. Any sad feelings usually go away within an hour; very rarely they may last a day or two. Studies have shown that most people feel a great sense of relief, happiness and contentment that lasts up to six months after they stop any regular writing.

Bullying

Being pressured to behave in a certain way, called names, teased, insulted, threatened, robbed or beaten up – are all forms of bullying. Bullies can be strangers, friends you've fallen out with, brothers or sisters, step-parents, parents, adults, or just the normal school variety. No one should have to put up with being bullied – it is one of the worst feelings in the world. Some people become severely frightened and depressed because they see no way out and don't tell anybody. They often feel that there is something the matter with them – that it is almost their own fault that they're being bullied. Their everyday lives are coloured with fear, nervousness and loss of self-esteem.

Girls talk more about their feelings and understand one another better, so they are in a better position to hurt one another by using a variety of more sophisticated forms of bullying apart from just fighting. They can suddenly give you the 'cold shoulder' and use criticism and 'psychological' techniques to make you feel bad, such as not accepting you into the group. You may have been friends with the bullies at some point, or even on some days, but they tease you, pick on you, or give you the cold shoulder perhaps because they're jealous and resentful of you, or because you won't join in something they're doing which you don't think is right – the reasons are endless.

Boarding schools can be particularly frightening because you are away from your parents and can even be trapped in your dormitory all night or weekend with people who bully you. You can feel you have no safe place to go and in some cases you can't even tell the prefect or monitor because they are the bully.

You may be worried that if you tell an adult you're being bullied somehow the bullies will find out and then you'll *really* get it. On the other hand, you may feel that you won't be believed, it won't be taken seriously, or that adults won't really know how to handle your problem effectively.

What To Do about Bullying

You must **take action**. If the bullying continues, it can have a long-term, horrible effect on you. You have a right to live without being picked on. Fortunately, a number of organizations, as well as schools and education authorities, are taking bullying far more seriously now. To start with, you or your parents can ring the **Anti-Bullying Campaign** helplines privately; they won't ask your name and won't tell anybody. They will be able to give you advice on exactly what you can do, as well as reacting with real understanding because they have probably been bullied themselves at one point.

Their numbers are: 071 378 1333/1177/7887/1188. Or you can send a stamped addressed envelope to:
Anti-Bullying Campaign, Room 37, 1st Floor, 6–10 Borough High Street, London, SE1 9QQ.

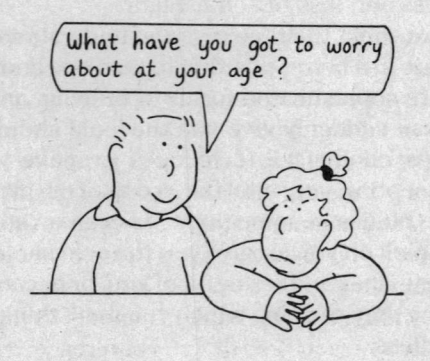

What have you got to worry about at your age?

Abuse

The term 'abuse' means different things to different people. For example, being emotionally abused can involve being denied love, neglected and hurt emotionally, while physical abuse can mean being hurt or injured. Sexual abuse, which has had the most publicity, involves a wide variety of things aside from adults touching your penis and vagina. The point is that if other people, whether they are young or adults, are doing things, saying things, or behaving in a way that makes you uncomfortable or unhappy or you don't feel is right – then you need to **talk** to someone about it. The person behaving in this way may be telling you to keep it secret, but as a child or teenager you have a **right** to be treated kindly and considerately by adults and those who care for you.

If this applies to you then it's essential to remember that it's not your fault. Tell an adult you feel safe with or you can ring Childline or the Samaritans (see page 79) or the **NSPCC Child Protection Line** free on 0800 800500. The NSPCC also produces helpful leaflets on abuse. Send a stamped addressed envelope to: **NSPCC**, 67 Saffron Hill, London EC1N 8RS or ring them on 071 242 1626.

Are You Gay?

Most boys fancy girls, *most* girls fancy boys. However, in every society, there are some boys who fancy boys, and some girls who fancy girls, and some who fancy both. For some of you, this may be a phase you are going through which you grow away from, but for others it is *not* a phase and they will *not* grow away from it.

There are many theories as to why a minority of people fancy their own sex. Many scientists now believe that this possibility is determined before you are even born – like being left-handed. In other words, fancying your own sex is no more 'wrong', 'sick', 'perverted' or 'sinful', than being left-handed. If that is how you feel, then that is how you feel. There is no reason whatsoever to feel guilty or ashamed in any way about this. However, by not being honest with *yourself* about your feelings, you could be doing yourself a lot of harm which could make you extremely miserable and seriously affect the rest of your life, even to the point of attempting suicide. Statistically, gay boys are more at risk from suicide than 'straight' boys. This seems to be because they feel terribly **alone** – that none of their friends are gay and that if their friends or family discovered the kind of feelings they were having, they would freak out. They feel they have no support and no one to approve of the way they feel. Perhaps they would feel better if they realised how many people in our society are gay. While pop stars and actors may be the most exposed professions for gay people to be identified in, there are gay people in *every* walk of life. There have been gay M.P.s, judges, gay boxers, top footballers and Wimbledon tennis champions.

What to Do

If you do fancy your own sex and you're confused, worried or unhappy about it for whatever reason, the first thing to do is to try to talk to your friends or family about the way you feel. You will probably be surprised to find that they will not freak out and will accept and support you. You can also ring several numbers for confidential and understanding advice and information, without giving your name. Or you can meet with groups of other people who feel the same way.

London Lesbian and Gay Switchboard, B M Switchboard, London, WC1N 3XX. Telephone 071 837 7234 (day or night). They can also refer you to local phone numbers.

Friend. Telephone 071 837 3337 (2 p.m. to 10 p.m. Monday and Tuesday, 7.30 p.m. to 10 p.m. Wednesday to Sunday). Counselling and support for gay people (boys and girls) and their relatives and friends.

Friend Women's Line. Telephone 071 837 2782 (7.30 p.m. to 10 p.m. Tuesday and Thursday).

Lesbian Line. Telephone 071 251 6911.

The Samaritans are listed in the front cover of your local telephone directory or ring Directory Enquiries. They will be happy to talk things over with you.

Childline Telephone 0800 1111.

Parental Problems

If your parents or the people who look after you are fighting between themselves, this can be very upsetting for you, not least because they are the very people you would naturally turn to to help you cope with unhappiness. Again, the solution is to try to talk to someone you feel comfortable with – a friend, an aunt, a teacher. If this is not enough or you cannot bring yourself to open up to someone you know, ring the Samaritans or Childline (see 'Who to Talk to').

If your parents or anyone in the house is drinking too much and this is worrying you, you can ring **Alcoholics Anonymous** on 071 403 0888 day or night. This is confidential and you don't need to give your name.

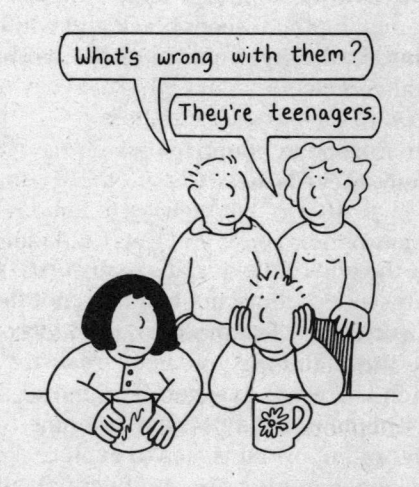

Chapter 7
The Way It Is

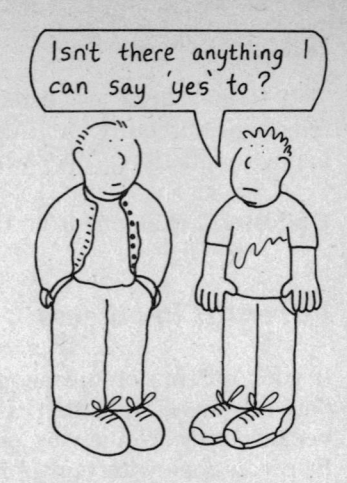

Isn't there anything I can say 'yes' to?

Many of you are probably sick and tired of being constantly told 'Say no to drugs', 'Say no to sex', 'Say no to drink', 'Say no to smoking'. It's not surprising that you feel this way when:

- You suspect your own parents may have said **'yes'** to these things when they were young (and may still be saying yes now that they are older).

- The media and health campaigns sensationalize and exaggerate these issues, making them seem black and white, completely safe or totally unsafe, the right choice or the wrong choice, the legal or the illegal choice.

- You see other European countries which have a completely different attitude to these issues.

Let's face it, at the end of the day, it's really up to you what you do with your body – not parents, not teachers, not the law, not the Archbishop of Canterbury. The problem is that in order to make decisions about these things, you need realistic and truthful information which is free of exaggeration, moral judgment and political policy. This is not always easy to come by and so I've selected a number of important issues to explore. You'll also find phone numbers you can ring for confidential, understanding advice, information and help without giving your name.

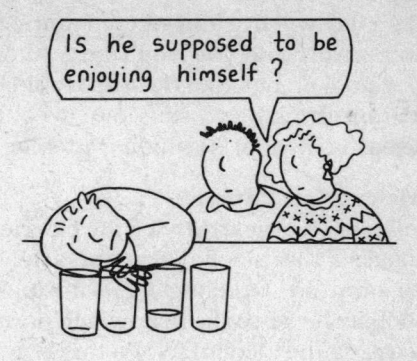

Alcohol

There isn't a week that goes by without some sensational 'drug bust' in the news. At the same time we are warned about Britain's 'drug epidemic'. However, we may suspect that something isn't quite right when we discover that one of Britain's most famous newsreaders, who has reported many drug stories, has himself been found by the police, face down in the gutter, out of his mind on booze! We also see photos in the newspapers of middle-aged politicians with a cigarette in one hand, a large glass of sherry in the other, sporting a nice dinner jacket and a lovely beer belly, going on about health and 'the evils of drug-taking'.

The truth of the matter is that Britain's most dangerous drug is not illegal. In fact it is advertised on the telly, your parents probably take it – it's alcohol. Legal or not, alcohol is the biggest danger that most of you will have to face.

Is Moderate Drinking Good for Your Health?

In our society, drinking is considered a 'comfortable', 'acceptable' way of socialising. In addition to this, the government receives a tremendous amount of money from the tax on alcohol – that's why drinking is not cheap. In fact going down the pub for a couple of pints each night can set you back by over £1,000 per year. Many adults believe that it is actually better for your health to drink 'moderately' than not to drink at all and this idea is reinforced by newspaper articles supporting this idea. However, while the media like to blow up reports that suggest that people who have one or two drinks a day will live longer, common sense should tell you that if this were really true, you would be getting a free glass of wine with every school dinner, and doctors would be ordering us to take up moderate drinking to save our lives! In addition to causing many diseases, alcohol is twice as fattening as pure sugar.

Why Alcohol Makes You Fatter
Gram for gram, alcohol has nearly twice the calories of sugar, but new research suggests that alcohol also drastically reduces your body's ability to burn fat. Drinking appears to slow down the body's fat metabolism because the liver which normally burns fat is too busy processing the alcohol. While this is going on, the fat that would have been burned, gets stored – usually in females' hips and thighs and in males' stomachs.

Boys Versus Girls
Women are increasingly becoming targets for advertisers of alcohol, but alcohol has special dangers for you females. We've always thought that females can't 'hold their drink' as well as males because they are smaller – in other words there is less of them to do the holding. However, it has recently been discovered that there is another important reason. Females have only about half as much of the enzyme *alcohol dehydrogenase* that breaks down alcohol in the stomach before it has a chance to pass through the stomach and enter the bloodstream. This is necessary to prevent you from getting really 'smashed' out of your head and giving yourself liver damage. So the way **one** drink affects a female is really equal to the way **two** drinks affect a male. The habit of men drinking a pint while women drink a half may be old-fashioned, but it's very sensible. Also women remain drunk for longer than men.

Can You Drown Your Sorrows with Drink?
No. In fact alcohol actually *depresses* your brain's activity in a way which is more likely to make you feel unhappy and depressed. Sorry.

One Thing at a Time
Mixing alcohol with other drugs, legal or not, could wind up killing you. (This even includes antihistamines.) Such a combination can

make you vomit in your sleep and because you are so 'drugged', you could breathe in the vomit and suffocate. Mixing these things also reduces your ability to breathe properly.

A Few Final Points About Alcohol

Addiction
Alcohol is a physically addictive drug producing withdrawal symptoms which can be fatal.

Violence
Drinking often leads to violence. Up to 50 per cent of murders involve alcohol, and when football fans are involved in rioting, they are often drunk.

Overdose and death
Drinking too much in one evening can kill you by alcohol poisoning. During 1987, for example, in England and Wales alone, 213 people dropped dead in a drunken stupor.

Brain Cells
Drinking kills them. An American study found that a large proportion of teenagers drink enough to affect their school performance. Most of them start early, before they have even turned 13.

Synergism
Alcohol seems to multiply the cancer-causing effects of smoking. For example, a person who smokes up to a packet of cigarettes a day, and doesn't drink, has a 52 per cent higher risk of oral cancer than a non-smoking non-drinker. But if he or she starts to have one drink a day, their risk goes up to 400 per cent! If they have more than two small drinks a day and smoke two packets of cigarettes their risk increases by fifteen times. It isn't clear why the risks of smoking and drinking 'synergise' in this way.

The point is that if you have no interest in drinking, don't bother taking up the habit. You shouldn't feel as if you're missing out on something and 'not able to enjoy yourself' without a drink. Don't be seduced by the idea that 'sensible drinking' is a natural part of growing up and that being a non-drinker is a bit extreme – because that's just what the brewers, distillers and their public relations firms want you to feel.

Help
If you are drinking often and don't feel you could give up, then do something about it now. If alcohol has become a crutch to lean on then you can ring **Alcoholics Anonymous**. Their number is in the phone book, or ring their main service number on 071 403 0888. You can also ring the **Samaritans**.

Smoking

While you probably hear all the time that smoking is dangerous, it is still worth pointing out some things you weren't aware of. Cigarette smoke contains a radioactive substance called *polonium 210*, and so for each year in which a person smokes a pack a day, they are exposing themselves to the same amount of radiation as if they had 200 chest X-rays.

By the way, about 410 people die prematurely each day from smoking-related diseases including cancer and heart disease – that's a jumbo jet a day! Some of these people didn't even smoke themselves but were merely exposed to other people's smoke over the years (passive smoking). If death by passive smoking were a sexually transmitted disease, the country would be up in arms about it.

Smoking and Your Body Shape
Girls are the most recent target for cigarette sales. Many of them think that smoking will help them stay slim. Surveys have even found that being worried about your weight can spur people to take up smoking as well as prevent them from giving it up. However, American scientists have found that the more cigarettes a person smokes, the more likely they are to develop a pot belly. Their body fat seems to settle around the waist and stomach.

Smoking Your Sex Life Away
While smoking has previously been linked to blocking the coronary (heart) arteries, a recent study published in the *American*

Journal of Urology found that smoking also damages the arteries in your penis that enable you to get an erection. This damage starts at a young age and can prevent you from having sex in a few years time, in which case it won't be a case of saying no to sex – because sex will say no to you!

Smoking and the Environment
In order to dry the tobacco to manufacture the cigarettes to sustain their habit, the average smoker requires a tree to be cut down every fortnight. As a result, 5 million hectares of land are chopped away every year. Tobacco farmers are also encouraged to use extra pesticides which make their way into the water supply. No doubt we'll see 'organically grown', 'green' brands of cigarette on the market soon!

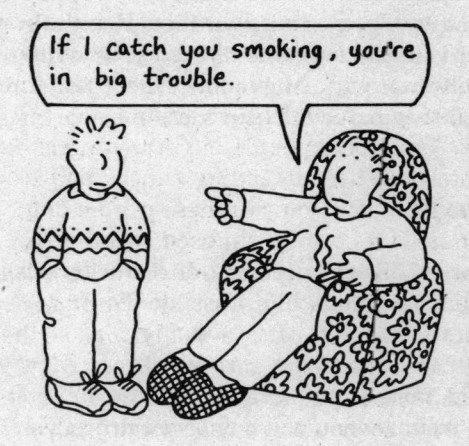

If I catch you smoking, you're in big trouble.

Puffing Parents
Studies have shown that if one of your parents smoke then you are more likely to take up smoking. Children whose parents smoke are three to four times more likely to end up in hospital with serious infectious diseases such as pneumonia, presumably because of the passive smoke they breathe in. 'Mainstream' smoke – the smoke inhaled by your parents from the butt end of a cigarette and then exhaled – may actually have *less* tar and nicotine than the 'sidestream' smoke drifting up from the hot end

of their lit cigarette, which you breathe in. Nearly 85 per cent of the smoke in a room is sidestream smoke. Now, assuming that you adore your parents and want them, as well as yourself, to live a long, healthy life, it's best to encourage them to quit by praising them for their efforts and success in cutting down or giving up. Showing them that you care is much more effective than simply nagging.

Help

If you want help stopping smoking, you can send a stamped address envelope to:
ASH 109 Gloucester Place, London W1H 3PH.
They can send you a 'giving up' pack. You can also ring Quitline on 071 487 3000. They provide advice and support and can also send you a 'giving up' pack. The Health Education Authority produces information on smoking – ring your local Health Promotion Unit. Their number is in the telephone directory, or write to the
H.E.A. Hamilton House, Mabledon Place, London WC1H 9TX Tel: 071 383 3833 (ask for the Information Department).

Dance Drugs

While the news is filled with sensational stories of all-night raves where people take things like Ecstasy (E) or LSD (Acid), few people seem to question who actually makes the drugs and whether you can actually be sure you'll get what you pay for. Unlike powerful prescription drugs sold by a chemist or administered in a hospital, when you buy dance drugs, you have no way of being sure what you're actually getting. One of the main problems with Ecstasy is being able to buy a real one. In Britain, people who have paid for Ecstasy, have instead been sold things like heroin and speed mixture, an LSD and 'speed' blend, or Ketamine – an anaesthetic drug used in surgical operations which has very unpleasant side effects. Of course, if you have a bad trip, you can't really write to the manufacturer and complain. When alcohol was illegal in America earlier this century, there were similar problems when people thought they were buying safely distilled booze on the black market. Just like those who manufacture cigarettes or booze, the people who make or distribute dance drugs are concerned with making a fat profit and not with your health.

If you want to know the real facts about any drugs without being preached to, told to 'say no to drugs' or given a lot of exaggerated, alarming information, contact:
Lifeline 101–103 Oldham Street, Manchester M4 1LW
Tel: 061 839 2054.
They also have a range of counselling services.

Using Your Nose

Sniffing glue, paint, lighter fluids, or breathing butane – known as *solvent abuse* – may seem an inexpensive, easy way to get out of your head. This is an easy way to kill yourself.

Spraying aerosol gases into your mouth can cause death by suffocation. Many of these substances can also cause you to choke to death on your own vomit or your heart to stop beating properly. Using plastic bags to breathe in solvents can also suffocate you. Many of the deaths from solvent abuse are due to the fact that the solvents affect your brain so quickly, that you are taken by surprise and are killed in some type of accident such as stepping in front of a car, falling or drowning. Long-term solvent abuse will leave you looking forward to permanent brain damage which will especially affect your ability to move. Sniffing petrol can give you lead poisoning, while aerosols and cleaning fluids can cause liver and kidney damage.

There is no 'good' side to solvent abuse. If you have tried it, stop now. If you find you can't stop, seek help **now**. You need it. For more confidential advice and information on solvent abuse ring **Resolve** on 0785 817885 or, write to: 30a High Street, Stone, Staffordshire ST15 8AW.

Sex

Your parents don't want you to have sex; your teachers, politicians, religious leaders and health authorities don't want you to have sex. Many of them have conveniently forgotten what it was like to be young themselves – they're obviously into more exciting things nowadays, like paying the mortgage and getting grey hair. In fact, it's actually illegal to have sex if you're under sixteen and if you're a gay male, the legal age is twenty-one, although this looks likely to drop to eighteen. However, despite all this, about 40 per cent of you under sixteen have already had sex and in the United States, where the authorities disapprove of sex even more, about 40 per cent of fourteen-year-olds have had sex. The point is that adults and governments can pass laws, lecture and educate you till they're blue in the face, but sex is such a private thing that it's obviously *you* who makes any sexual decisions – whether *they* like it or not. Therefore, it's you who has the responsibility of knowing more about preventing or dealing with some of the problems that sometimes come with sex. If you're having sex or think you might be in the near future, learn about contraception now. Nowadays you can get excellent confidential advice about contraception, as well as free contraceptives which are easily available. The details are available under the section 'Help' on the opposite page. Without giving you a lecture on sex education and contraception here are a few things you may not have been aware of.

Emergency Contraception
If you are a girl who has had full sex within the last three days without using any form of contraception, forgot your pill, or used a condom which leaked and you are now worried you might be pregnant, you can get a form of contraceptive tablet that you take within seventy-two hours *after* the time you had sex, which will prevent you from getting pregnant. You can also have an intra-uterine device (IUD) fitted within five days after the time you had sex – that will prevent pregnancy. So, if you are worried, don't sit around blaming yourself or worrying, **act now** (see below).

Are You Pregnant?
If you are worried that you are pregnant because you had full sex with no contraception, or you used a condom which leaked, and your period is now late, then the first thing is to find out if you really are pregnant – just being worried can make your period late. Get a pregnancy test – you can either do this secretly by buying a

do-it-yourself urine test at the chemist or you can have the chemist do a test for you. You can also have a free pregnancy test done (see below). The important thing is **do not delay** finding out the truth.

You ARE Pregnant
If you are pregnant, **do not** torture yourself with guilt and worry – you are certainly not alone. For example, there are close to 200,000 abortions a year in Britain. The important thing is to realize there is a lot of free, confidential help and advice now available and **your parents will not be told**. Nowadays, if you are up to nine weeks pregnant (that is, nine weeks since the first day of your last period) there is a tablet available from certain clinics which will stop the pregnancy from developing. It is called RU486 and it will require several visits to the clinic. Many girls stay at home worrying and don't ask for help until they are twelve weeks pregnant – that is too late. **Act now** – the sooner you speak to someone confidentially the better you will feel, and you do not need to give your name. There are helplines and kind sympathetic people who can help you decide what you want to do. There is even a pre-recorded computerized phone line you can ring for practical information and you simply listen to the voice but don't have to speak to anybody. Again, **please don't leave it** (see 'Help' below).

Help
For twenty-four-hour pre-recorded computerized information on free emergency contraception, pregnancy tests, unwanted pregnancy, abortion or general contraception, ring: **Brook Helpline** on 071 617 8000. For someone to talk to on these topics or if you want to see someone about any of these things, ring:
The Brook Advisory Centre Central Office on 071 708 1234, or **The Family Planning Association Central Office** on 071 636 7866 (9 a.m. to 5 p.m. Monday to Friday, 4.30 p.m. on Friday).

Your own doctor is likely to be very helpful and is unlikely to tell your parents, but if you don't want to see him or her, you can secretly ring another GP (look under 'doctors' in the Yellow Pages), ask the receptionist if they provide confidential help for under sixteens (if you are) on the particular matter and you should be able to see the GP without anyone else knowing. If the receptionist doesn't seem very helpful then ring another GP. Boys and girls can also get free packs of condoms from all of the above sources.

If you are concerned about sexually transmitted diseases you can go to any special clinic. You normally don't need an appointment, and you can find them by ringing your local hospital and asking for the nearest 'special clinic'.

For confidential advice and counselling on AIDS and HIV infection ring the free National AIDS Helpline on 0800 567123 (twenty-four hours), or Terence Higgins Trust Helpline on 071 242 1010 (3 p.m. to 10 p.m. daily).

Sexually Transmitted Diseases (STDs)

AIDS has received a tremendous amount of publicity as the most dangerous disease which can be sexually transmitted. Because of this, many people have overlooked more ordinary STDs that have killed even more people. In the ten years between 1982 and 1992, for example, eighty-nine women in Britain died from AIDS which they got through sex (by the way, fifty-six of these women were from other countries, or had lived in countries where AIDS was much more common). At the same time, many more women died or were damaged by other STDs, such as those described below.

Genital Warts

These are caused by *human papilloma viruses (HPV)* of which there are over sixty different types. Three of these HPVs have been linked to cancer of the cervix, vagina and possibly the penis, and usually cause an invisible infection which only a doctor can detect. Fortunately, the HPVs that cause most genital warts don't seem to be linked to cancer.

Chlamydia

A bacterial infection, this is the most common STD. About 75 per cent of infected females have no symptoms. Chlamydia is the primary cause of pelvic inflammatory disease, which can scar the fallopian tubes and possibly prevent women from being able to have children in future. About 75 per cent of infected males will have symptoms. About one in ten sexually active people have chlamydia each year, however it is easily curable with antibiotics.

Hepatitis B
Hepatitis B is a risk for gay males who have unprotected intercourse. Half of those people infected develop acute hepatitis and up to 10 per cent of infected people become chronic carriers who may develop cirrhosis of the liver or liver cancer. There is an effective vaccine available from your GP to prevent Hepatitis B.

Check It Out
The point of all of this is that if you have any unusual symptoms in or around your penis or vagina, have it checked out. Don't wait for it to go away by itself, because if you have become infected it could go 'silent' – making you think it's gone away when it hasn't. Also, if you're just worried that you may have been exposed to an STD you may find it reassuring to have a chat with someone. You can talk to someone or be examined, without giving your real name, your parents will not be told, and you usually don't even need an appointment. If you find that you do have an STD you certainly have **no reason to feel guilty** or 'dirty', as a huge proportion of the population has had, or will get, some form of STD at one point or another. In America for example there are twelve million new STD cases each year.

The other thing to mention is that condoms are an excellent form of protection from most STDs, and you can get a variety of different types free. Those containing *nonoxynol-9* are even more protective against many different germs.

Masturbation
A comedian once wrote: '99 per cent of men masturbate and 1 per cent are liars' (although the percentage may be a bit lower for women). Just in case any of you are feeling guilty or ashamed of masturbating, it's important to realize that masturbation is not only normal and natural, it is actually good for you. Apart from obviously feeling good, you also learn how your 'equipment' works and it makes you more sexually confident and comfortable about your body. Boys can also learn how to put condoms on

correctly. This is important. At one major pregnancy clinic they asked the boyfriends of the pregnant girls, who claimed that they used a condom but it broke, to show, using a fake willie, how they actually put on the condom. The clinic found that 50 per cent of the boys failed to put the condoms on properly – some were inside out, others not unrolled fully! They now recommend that practice makes perfect.

Finally, it has to be said that whenever you are told about some aspect of sex, it's usually some sort of warning about risks and danger of one sort or another. It must make sex sound like some sort of grim gamble – a necessary 'evil' that should be kept to an absolute minimum. But if you think about it, if sex really were that bad, people wouldn't keep doing it, would they? The truth is that, as with many other enjoyable things in life, you should simply be smart about it. On the other hand, if you don't want to have sex, you needn't feel you have to – at the end of the day the choice is yours.

Sanitary Protection

The manufacturers of sanitary protection spend millions of pounds each year trying to get you to spend your money on their products. They even go so far as to suggest the use of panty liners all month long even when you're not menstruating. The implication being that there is something 'dirty' about your normal vaginal secretions – this is complete **rubbish**, and besides, what are pants for anyway?

They have also given talks at schools about the benefits of using panty liners and tampons rather than sanitary towels, trying to hook you while you're young. This gives a false impression, because tampons are certainly not any healthier than sanitary towels and can even be unhealthy if not used with care.

There are all manner of sanitary towels and tampons available on the market – different shapes and sizes, different absorbencies, different ways of fitting – and the only way to find out which suits you best is to try them. Sometimes you may be able to get sample packs, or you could buy a pack and divide them between a few friends to check them out before you decide whether they suit you. Once you find one that suits your level of flow and is comfortable and easy to use, stick with it. As your flow varies through your period, you may use two or even three different types.

Some girls find that tampons are easier and more comfortable than sanitary towels. If you decide to use them, you should be aware that it is essential to use them properly otherwise they can cause some unpleasant problems.

Firstly, always use an appropriate absorbency for the particular day of your period, the lower the better. Change them regularly and never leave them in for more than about four hours at a time. Don't leave them in overnight; use a sanitary towel instead. In fact, it is better to alternate with sanitary towels during your period. Modern sanitary towels are easily hidden and are very efficient. Because the chemicals used to manufacture some tampons are thought by scientists to be absorbed into the body, use non-chlorine bleached tampons.

If you do not use tampons sensibly, you are asking for trouble. Because it is unnatural to leave things like tampons in your vagina, they have been found to cause unnatural vaginal dryness, or even peeling of the lining of the vagina, leading to tiny ulcers. Also, the fibres from tampons can become embedded in the lining of the vagina causing serious inflammation.

One particular serious, although fortunately rare, side-effect of misusing tampons is known as *toxic shock syndrome*, and younger women have a much higher risk of contracting TSS than older women. The early symptoms are flu-like and include a temperature about 39°C, vomiting, diarrhoea, a sore throat, aching muscles, a headache and stiff and tender neck, dizziness and fainting, a rash especially on the hands, feet and body. After this, symptoms become more severe and can even be fatal. Many women are thought to be suffering from milder forms of TSS which can recur. If you have any TSS symptoms – and they do not always all appear – remove your tampon and consult your doctor. For information, send a stamped addressed envelope to:
The Women's Environmental Network, Aberdeen Studios, 22 Highbury Grove, London N5 2EA.

Chapter 8
Improving Exam Performance

Exam-taking is a particular skill that some people will naturally be better at than others. It is really only one of several ways to judge your achievement in school – and is not necessarily the best or fairest way. Most schools will use a combination of techniques, such as exams, project work and general assessment. Unfortunately, however, exams are almost always part of the process.

Taking exams is much more than simply an 'intellectual' performance. 'Using your brain' means making sure it is operating under the best conditions possible – this is usually overlooked by most people and this is where there's room for improvement. Let's consider the demands placed upon your brain at exam time.

Memory and Learning
Exams require you not only to absorb information but to understand its full meaning and then to recall that information during the exam.

Concentration
Concentration is absolutely necessary to be able to absorb information to begin with, so you have to be able to remain alert while studying, listening to teachers (terribly sorry), and taking the exam itself.

Thinking Quickly and Clearly
This is vital in order to put the information you remember in the right place and to organize yourself quickly enough to finish the exam in time.

The 'Big Vision'
You can't just churn out facts and figures, names and dates. For better grades you have to show that you have a general understanding – an overview of a subject.

Being Selective
By the time your exam arrives you are probably suffering from information overload. Therefore you must be able to select the most important bits of information from all the less relevant bits in order to provide a good answer.

Creativity
The best exam answers often come from thinking in creative and abstract ways. This shows that you are capable of seeing things from a different angle to others and aren't simply churning out a textbook answer.

Stress
Becoming over worried or nervous competes with the other demands placed on your brain during an exam and can reduce your performance.

Planning Your Attack

Dull as it may sound, you really have to try and plan your approach to exams – in some cases like training for an athletic event.

Prediction
Try to predict the general types of questions. The first place to start is simply to ask your teachers what type of exam questions are likely to come up. Remember, it's in their interest that you do well or else it makes them look like poor teachers.

Set Priorities
Some people try to study everything. Instead choose the most likely topics and focus on these. This is particularly important if you've left it too late, and there's little chance of covering all areas anyway.

Study with Friends
Misery loves company and you're also more likely to understand and absorb information if you discuss it with someone. You can also mix business with pleasure to make studying a less boring experience. Some people don't have photographic memories and studying by talking about the subject may help them to absorb the topic more effectively than staring at a page.

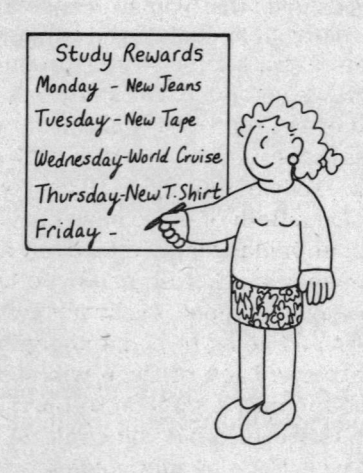

Reward Yourself
To keep yourself going list some things or activities you want to do if you complete a certain amount of studying. Better yet, get your parents to provide the rewards!

Mock Exams
These can be a good way of both clarifying your thoughts about the topics you've studied, sharpening your exam technique and reducing the fear of the real exam.

Study in Short Bursts
Don't study for more than four or five hours a day – there's no extra benefit. It's what, how and when you study that's important.

While there's obviously no substitute for studying, the following advice will help you make the most of what you've learned and enable you to perform at your best come exam time.

Body Clocks and Sleep

Our bodies and minds are programmed by a small group of brain cells (our body clock) to run on a particular schedule. Mental and physical abilities change dramatically throughout a twenty-four-hour day. For example, the ability to work with our hands, concentration, and memory, reaches a peak in the afternoon and falls to a low in the middle of the night. In fact the only thing that improves at night is hormone production – you produce most of your growth hormone while you sleep. The study of how your body and mind are affected by the time of day is called *chronobiology*.

Our body clocks are set and kept on time by daylight, which also keeps us alert. The study of how light affects your mind and body is called *photobiology*. Both of these newer sciences have taught us a few things about thinking more effectively and feeling better.

Confusing your body clock will make you less alert and less effective. A good way to confuse it is by not getting enough sleep or enough daylight and going to bed and getting up at different times on different days. Lack of sleep will still enable a tennis player to play good tennis, a surgeon to operate successfully, a pilot to land a jet. However, what you **can't** do is read a book or remember things well. For example, soldiers with little sleep can shoot accurately but can't remember things like topping up their hip flasks with water.

- Research has found that young people need nine and a half hours sleep or more, particularly during exam time. If you need an alarm clock to wake you up every morning then you are not getting enough sleep.

- You should sleep at regular times so as not to confuse your body clock.

IMPROVING EXAM PERFORMANCE

- Taking a short nap (twenty minutes or so) during the afternoon dip will also help you study and perform better ... just make sure you don't fall asleep during your exam!

- You must get enough daylight. This means studying in a well-lit room, preferably near a window. Whenever possible, take breaks outdoors.

Your brain has certain 'prime times' when it is more effective.

- The best times to study are (if for example you get up at 7.00 a.m.) between 9.00 a.m. and 12.00 noon, and then late afternoon between 4.00 and 6.00 p.m. These times are only approximate and I also realise that many of you can't study at these times because you're in school or working.

- The worst times to study are usually after lunch, because your body clock goes into a dip between around 1.00 to 3.00 p.m., and also at night. Usually, the later it gets, the less effective your studying will be, so if you have to study in the evening do it early.

- Although some people claim that they are more creative after 11.00 p.m., please remember that GCSEs take place during the day. Studying late at night will disrupt your body clock and anyway, you won't learn as well at night.

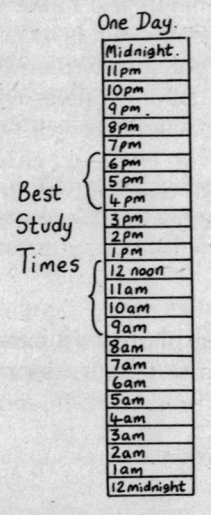

One Day.

Midnight
11pm
10pm
9pm
8pm
7pm
6pm
5pm
4pm
3pm
2pm
1pm
12 noon
11am
10am
9am
8am
7am
6am
5am
4am
3am
2am
1am
12 midnight

Best Study Times: 4pm–6pm and 9am–12 noon

Exercise

We are led to believe that there are two opposite types of students: the fit, Arnold Swarzenegger-type whose thick neck matches his IQ; and the wimpy nerd, who's a bookworm and wears thick glasses. However, in reality, students who remain fit generally do better in school. Furthermore, recent studies have found that twenty minutes of aerobic-type exercise will **immediately:**

- improve performance on IQ-type tests
- reduce feelings of stress
- improve altertness and concentration
- help you think more quickly and clearly
- improve memory and learning
- make you think more creatively.

Aerobic exercise doesn't just mean running round a wet sports field in the cold. It includes any exercise which makes your heart beat fast and your rate of breathing increase. This means any activity which uses large groups of muscles, especially in the legs, for example skating, jogging, skipping rope, fast walking, cycling, swimming – even dancing to one side of an LP or cassette. The key is to get your heart rate and breathing up and to keep it there for at least twenty minutes. When you do this, your brain releases endorphins which affect the way you think and feel. The endorphin 'high' you get from this will immediately improve your creative abilities and decision making. (See Chapter 9 on how this works.)

- Between now and your exam, try to do some type of aerobic exercise at least three times a week. (As exercise peps you up, it's best not to do it too near bedtime, or you could have trouble falling asleep.)

- On the day of your exam, if possible, exercise before your exam starts, preferably outdoors. This is especially helpful for afternoon exams, when you are likely to be more sluggish.

Nutrition

Blood Sugar

The amount of your body's own glucose that circulates around your bloodstream, your blood sugar, has to remain at an acceptable level. If the level dips, which can happen when you try to diet or skip a meal, you may become more forgetful, less able to make decisions, more tired and even depressed or aggressive and 'edgy'. Your brain cells actually run on glucose in order to work properly. However, by eating or drinking things which contain sugar, your brain can actually end up with *less* sugar, leaving you feeling sluggish and less able to think clearly! This is because your body makes its own sugars from the normal foods you eat and it over-reacts to outside sugars by actually lowering the level of sugar which normally circulates in your bloodstream – the exact opposite of what you might expect. Eating sugar also increases the amount of insulin you produce which may cause your brain to produce a natural sleeping substance – *serotonin* – making you less alert. (See 'Sugar, Glucose and "Quick Energy"' in Chapter 4 and 'Sports Drinks and "Energy Giving" Products' in Chapter 9.)

Caffeine

Caffeine is found in coffee and tea but it's also contained in cola and other soft drinks, chocolate and of course 'stay awake' pills. While caffeine may give you a quick lift, the effect is very short lived and you can end up with even lower blood sugar levels, feeling worse than when you started. This is especially so when you combine caffeine with sugary things as in cola drinks or sugared tea and coffee. Caffeine also raises the levels of two important stress hormones and can make people very jittery and nervous.

- Before you study and on the day of your exam, avoid all sugar things including glucose sports drinks, dextrose or glucose tablets and sweets – don't believe advertising claims.

- Avoid caffeine between now and your exam. However, if you regularly drink tea or coffee do not suddenly give it up on the day of your exam or you will get withdrawal symptoms, such as a headache, which will only make matters worse.

- It is a complete myth that starving yourself will make you peform better in an exam. Eat breakfast before the exam and eat regularly to keep your blood sugar level stable.

- While eating complex carbohydrates (starches, such as pasta, rice, potatoes, bread) is good and necessary for maintaining blood sugar, eating a lot of these at lunch immediately before your exam begins could make you sleepier. Remember, your body clock may make you a bit sluggish anyway during the afternoon.

Although there have been claims by vitamin manufacturers that taking their special (and expensive) vitamin tablets will make children more intelligent, scientists think this is complete nonsense and a waste of money. Eating a well-balanced diet will give you a much better vitamin supply than tablets.

Alcohol, Antihistamines and Cannabis

All of these make you less alert. Alcohol kills brain cells and some antihistamines make you very dozy. Don't use them while you're studying or the night before your exam. If you need medication, for hay fever for example, ask your GP or chemist about antihistamines which don't cause drowsiness. If you have a cold or flu, don't take the night-time cold remedies which make you sleep better as they contain alcohol and other drugs which give you a terrible hangover and you won't think as clearly on the day of your exam.

TV, Radio and Music

Whatever you might think, studying with the TV on will affect your ability to absorb the things you're trying to learn. The same goes for background music which you love so much that it may compete for your attention, particularly if it has lots of interesting lyrics which may be much more exciting than the page in front of you. If you must listen, choose music you find pleasant, not amazing. Party afterwards. By the way, recent experiments have found that, after watching television, many people feel less alert and have more difficulty concentrating. A recent survey by the US Education Department found that pupils who watched the least amount of television had significantly higher reading scores than pupils who watched most.

Stress and Worry

Stress appears to be hitting people at younger and younger ages because of the more complicated and competing demands being placed on them. Our society, more than ever, is pushing the importance of success, achievement, winning, being number one. Television forces more and more images of 'poor boy made good' – modern-day rags to riches stories – in our face. The bottom line is that on the one hand people may feel they have more opportunities than their parents, while on the other hand they feel they must take these opportunities and succeed more than ever. We're made to believe that the more successful job you have the happier you will be – a one to one ratio. A dustman is much, much more unhappy than a brain surgeon or a movie actor. This is simply **not true**.

The point is that you have to put your exams in the right perspective. Just think about the task at hand – doing the best you can. Don't waste time and worry (which will only make your exams harder) thinking about the *consequences* of your exam results – what secondary school or university will I go to? What kind of job will I get? How much money will I earn? Will my parents approve of my results?

One of the advantages of being young is not having to worry as much about such monumental eventualities as adults do. Unfortunately, you are often being robbed of this advantage. In addition to this, your life will not be destroyed by one exam result, however poor. Most exams can be taken again and there are other ways you can make up for a poor result. Don't lose sight of the overall picture.

If you feel that your parents have unrealistic expectations for you and are placing too much pressure on you to succeed, tell them this if you can. You may find it a help to show them this section. If you can't, either because they won't hear any of it or you don't feel able to, then ask a relative or family friend or brother or sister or several of them to explain this to your parents. Someone at school, a teacher you like, a guidance counsellor, even the head could stick his nose in and reason with them. Parents should be aware that they issue approval and disapproval, often without saying the words, even without knowing they're doing it.

Chapter 9
Getting Physical

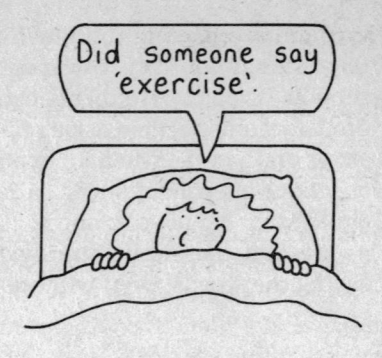

What can exercise do for you? It can give you better results at school; improve your self-confidence, lift depression and reduce stress; make you better looking, more creative and energetic; lower your body fat, improve your immune system and make you less tired; and make you better with the opposite sex.

You might think that these are wild claims, but recent scientific experiments have shown that exercise *will* achieve these things. Unlike make-up, clothes or food or slimming aids, exercise is difficult to package and sell as a product in a high street shop. Apart from anything else, it is basically *free*, something you can do for yourself. For this reason, advertisers would rather spend their millions pushing their new trainers, rather than spelling out the benefits of the exercise you get from running in them.

Exercise has had a terrible image – running around a wet sports field in the cold, huffing and puffing by numbers, or competitive or team sports such as football, hockey or volleyball – which many of us hate. But things are already changing for the better. In fact the term 'exercise' should be changed to *physical activity* and this can include, for example, dancing, roller skating, fast walking, cycling, skate boarding, or simply mucking about with a football or frisbee. The fact is, that humans were built to be active and if we are not, then we'll be *less* healthy, happy, good looking and intelligent.

How It Works

Exercise causes your brain and spinal cord to produce their own powerful opium-related drugs called *endorphins*. If you were caught selling a powdered version of these hard drugs on a street corner, you'd be busted and sent to prison for a long time. Endorphins are 'mood-altering' drugs which produce a 'high' after about twenty minutes of aerobic-type exercise. This isn't surprising if you stop and think about it, as your body has to be able to produce natural painkillers. Back in the caveman days, chasing animals to eat or fighting for survival was a painful business. Nature also has to provide you with some sort of immediate reward for doing something which is good for you, but may feel a bit exhausting at first. Long-distance runners are so experienced at achieving a 'runner's high', that merely expecting it appears to stimulate their own endorphin production. And when they actually do run, the combination of low-level pain and constant rhythm seems to cause a 'global activation' of opium compounds in their central nervous systems which give them an amazing feeling after, and sometimes during, a run. The high lasts between thirty minutes and five hours. This is probably one reason why people enjoy dancing until they're tired and sweaty – lots of aerobic movement and a hard steady beat.

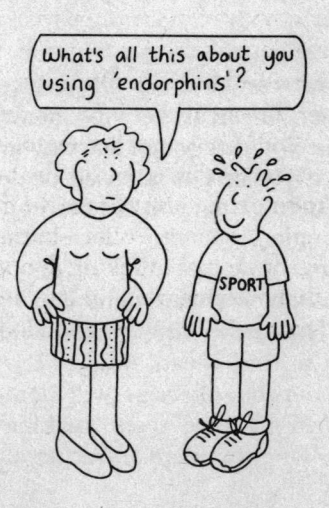

The Psychological Benefits

These chemicals, as well as other changes in your brain chemistry, are responsible for a whole variety of psychological benefits that you probably weren't aware of.

Sexier
Studies have found that exercise makes people feel more attractive and more self-confident when it comes to dealing with the opposite sex. (In fact, exercise generally raises your self-esteem and improves your self-image in a variety of other ways as well.) If you give off these vibes, other people actually *do* see you as more attractive. Studies have also shown that people often feel more 'romantically inclined' shortly after aerobic exercise.

Happier
Exercise can also make you happier. In the United States, exercise is now being used in many hospitals as an official treatment for child, teenage or adult depression. It lifts people's moods and makes them more optimistic. This is often 'prescribed' for the morning, when depression tends to be at its worst. Doing sports or exercise with others may also help you to take your mind off your problems and give you a sense of accomplishment – focusing on the here and now as opposed to other worries.

Stress
Stress and nervousness are dramatically reduced by the chemical effects of exercise. Physical activity neutralizes the stress hormones that make you jittery and leaves you feeling more well balanced. So even if you're not stressed or depressed, exercise will make you feel better than you did before.

Better Results
Better grades at school and in exams can result from regular exercise. Exercise has now been linked with doing better at school. In addition to this, recent studies have found that only twenty minutes of aerobic exercise will **immediately** improve your performance in IQ type tests, making you think more creatively and improving your concentration, alertness and speed.

(For more information see Chapter 8.) It is thought that aerobic activity affects the way brain cells function, resulting in greater intellectual performance.

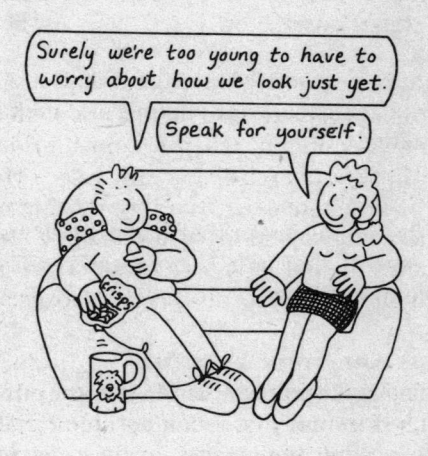

The Physical *Benefits*

We all know that exercise can build muscles, burn up calories and prevent heart disease but there are other more interesting things it can achieve.

Energy
Exercise gives you more energy. Contrary to popular belief, exercise actually peps you up. In fact, this is one reason you shouldn't exercise before bedtime. Exercising around lunch time can make you more alert in the afternoon (if you want to be, that is).

Improved Immune System
People who exercise have been found to have more *natural killer cells (NK cells)* which patrol the bloodstream and kill foreign invading germs. One study found that unfit people have colds that last about three times longer than fit people. All this may sound odd, but as with endorphins, nature had to protect people from infection. When people ran it was usually away from something,

and they were likely to cut themselves in the process, so when people ran, the body automatically increased its immunity against germs to prevent the cuts from becoming infected – remember, there were no chemists around in those days.

Better Looking
Exercise can make you better looking because it will change your body shape, your muscles, your posture and make you healthier and more attractive.

Bullying
Boys who are fit-looking are probably less likely to be a target for bullying, and even if they are, their greater self-esteem makes them more able to cope with it.

Aerobic versus Anaerobic Exercise
Most of the benefits discussed so far come from doing aerobic exercises which does not just mean aerobic classes. It involves any continuous-action movements using large muscle groups: dancing, fast walking, roller or ice skating, cycling and so on all fall into this category. The information below will give you more suggestions. Aerobic activity makes you breathe faster and your heart pump faster. This results in making your heart, circulatory system, lungs and muscles far more efficient; it also makes you burn fat supplies to give you energy.

Menu of Aerobic Exercises
Dancing
Skateboarding
Table tennis
Cutting grass (using pushmower)
Hockey
Aerobic dancing
Step aerobics
Tennis
Raquetball
Squash
Rollerskating
Ice skating

Cycling
Stationary cycling
Football
Basketball
Swimming
Treading water (fast)
Rowing (or rowing machine)
Downhill skiing
Cross Country skiing
Walking
Running
Golf (if you walk the course)
Skipping (using a skipping rope)

Anaerobic exercise is very much the opposite, requiring short bursts of intense energy as in weight training, sprinting, and some calisthenics such as sit-ups that are designed to strengthen specific muscles. Energy for this comes mainly from your own sugar supplies stored within your muscles.

Fat-Burning Exercises

It's important first to dispel a few myths about exercise, body shape and weight.

Spot reduction involves diets, exercise or electronic muscle stimulators which claim to remove fat from certain parts of your body, such as your hips, thighs or stomach. Rubbish! Doing hundreds of sit-ups, for example, may strengthen your stomach muscles but will do nothing to remove a pot belly. The reason is that fat is not burned in the area that you are exercising. For instance, running doesn't necessarily burn fat on the legs; fat may be burned on your back or face, and your blood will deliver this fat energy to your leg muscles where it's needed most. The way your body stores fat in certain areas is part of your general body shape, which is inherited. Trying to isolate specific areas alone for flubber removal is a complete nonsense. However, by eating in a healthy, low-fat way (see Chapter 4) and keeping physically active, you can lose fat in the areas you want – as well as in some other areas. Remember your body tries to protect its fat supplies.

For girls, this means hips, thighs and bottom; for boys, stomach. If you try a fast weight-loss programme, your body will hang on to this fat – and you are likely to lose it in these places last and regain it there first, and you will probably end up fatter in the long run (see Chapter 3).

If you start exercising as recommended below, you will become slimmer and firmer but you may not actually lose weight and may even *gain* a little. This is good and is due to the fact that your excess fat is being replaced by muscle, which is smaller in size, but heavier than the old blubber. Another reason why weighing yourself can be very misleading.

The key to the activities which achieve a healthier and more attractive body shape and composition are simple.

- Ensure you do at least twenty minutes of good quality aerobic activity at least three times a week – preferably more. This means getting your heart rate and breathing up and keeping it there.

- People who are aerobically fit are found to have more fat-burning compartments inside their muscle cells. This keeps them burning fat a lot of the time and means that if they continue to eat the same as they always did, they're likely to burn more calories than they take in. Even if they eat more calories (often the case with men who exercise) they'll still have burned more than they ate. In addition to this, aerobic activity seems to have a positive effect on your body's appetite control mechanism, which can be weakened by an inactive lifestyle. You are also more likely to make more intelligent food choices because your body will automatically set nutritional priorities to replace lost nutrients by making you eat healthier foods.

- Muscle is a 'hungry' tissue: 450 grams of muscle burns thirty to fifty calories a day just doing nothing, while the same weight of body fat burns only two. So the more muscle you have, the more calories and fat you burn just sitting down in a classroom. This is precisely why building a bit more muscle will help you keep your fat down and improve your body shape.

- Some research has suggested that obese people who have trouble losing weight, appear to have too many 'fast' anaerobic-type muscle fibres and not enough 'slow' aerobic-type muscle fibres. It may therefore be better for them to concentrate purely on the aerobic types of activities.

- Just keeping active on a regular basis, however, is extremely helpful (such as walking instead of being driven, doing gardening or household chores instead of being a couch potato). Over six months, the amount of activity you engage in does add up.

By the way, exercise should not become a new, more 'acceptable' form of diet addiction or eating disorder. Obsessive concern with weight, shape and exercise is not healthy. Girls who lose too much body fat will face serious risks to their feminine appearance and to their general health (see Chapter 3). Exercise is intended simply to make people healthier and the side-effect will be a better body shape.

Muscle Strengthening

The strength and stamina of your muscles are increased by exercises that give *resistance* to particular movements. You can achieve this in several ways.

Calisthenics
Exercises such as press-ups or sit-ups, are the most basic and convenient method, since you lift your own body weight and need no equipment.

Isometric Exercises
These can be done at any time, anywhere. You tense your muscles against a fixed object such as a doorway or a wall or against each other. These require little movement, no equipment and only take a number of seconds to do. Their drawback is that they only work the muscle at one limited angle.

Partner Routines
Working with a partner is good at making exercises more fun, adding motivation, friendly competition and companionship,

because you can do them with a friend or relative. Your partner provides the resistance.

Water Calisthenics

Exercises in water use the water's resistance, require little space even in a crowded pool, and those who can't swim can also do them. You can do them by yourself, with a partner and there are often classes at your local pool.

Weight Training

The best way to increase strength is by working out with weights. This can be done by everybody – not just bodybuilders who are an extreme example of training with very heavy weights. You shouldn't be doing weight training if you're under nine as your joints and bones are developing very rapidly and could be adversely affected. At any age, you should only lift weights under the guidance of an experienced trainer who will control the weight you lift and the way you lift it. A good programme for overall fitness will include about ten to twelve exercises, half for your upper body, half for your lower body. Most importantly it must be scheduled so that each muscle has at least a full day's rest before you exercise it again. Exercising the same muscle two days in a row will make it weaker not stronger because you won't give it time to recover and rebuild itself. So either exercise different muscles on different days (for example, upper body one day, lower body the next) or leave a couple of days between workouts.

Circuit Training

You can add a bit of aerobic benefit to strength training by doing several repetitions of an exercise and then moving quickly on to the next exercise with only a fifteen to thirty second rest, at most, between exercises. This can involve weights and calisthenics and enables you to work on stomach, arms, legs, hips and back in rapid succession. This is usually done in a gym with other people.

Variable Resistance Machines

A new generation of variable resistance machines are even better than normal weights at isolating and strengthening muscles. They are normally found at health clubs and gyms because they are big and expensive.

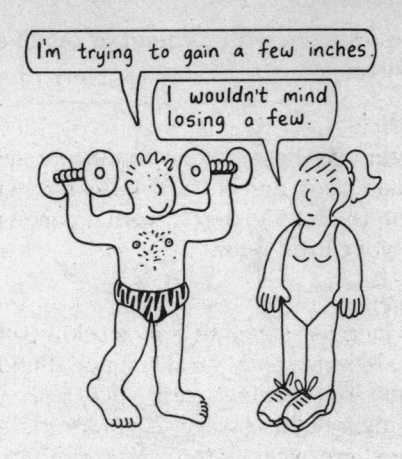

Keeping Interested in Physical Activity

Half of all people who start exercising, drop out within six months. You mustn't think of physical activity as an 'exercise campaign', activity must become a natural part of your lifestyle like brushing your teeth or watching television, which stays with you for life. Here are some pointers to help stay physical.

Variety
Doing the same type of exercises all the time can be extremely boring. There is a large menu of activities to choose from – dancing one day, cycling the next, swimming the day after etc. Make use of this variety as this type of cross training will make you even more fit than sticking to the same boring routine.

Join Other People
Activity in a group, class or with a partner is far more likely to keep you at it and you'll work harder as well. If you promise people you'll join them you're less likely to let them down than if it's left purely to you to do the activity. Form your own casual group to do some activity after school, evenings or weekends.

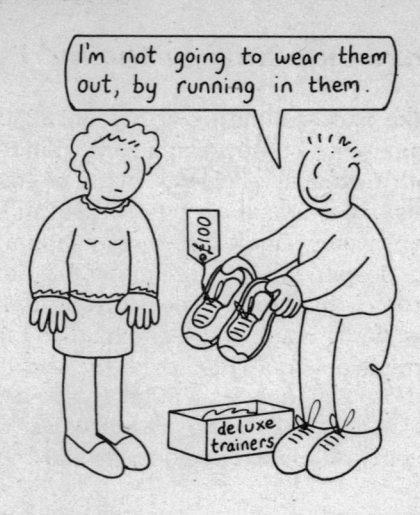

Plan a Visit
Arrange to meet someone some distance away and run, walk, cycle, rollerskate or skateboard there. When you do meet up, instead of always sitting and chatting, go for a walk and blabber away on foot.

Convenience
Find convenient times and easy to reach places – even school – otherwise you'll find excuses not to do any activity.

Use PE Classes to Your Advantage
If you have to attend them, make the best use of them. If you don't like competitive sports ask your PE teacher if you and others can do some other form of exercise or activity – show your teacher this chapter.

Create Your Own Menu
Stick your own menu on the wall, which includes all the possible activities mentioned in this chapter, all the possible people, places, times and ways you can do any of these activities. This way you should be able to choose something to do a few times a week, without having to think too hard.

Sports Drinks and 'Energy Giving' Products

The sports drinks market alone is worth a cool £200 million a year. During a hot summer, you buy around 1¼ million cans a week. Thanks to a lot of expensive adverts, many of you believe these products will make you more energetic, or will quench your thirst better than plain water. Don't waste your money because they won't. In fact, despite all the technobabble about 'glucose', 'dextrose', 'isotonic', 'hypotonic', 'electrolytes' etc. – these drinks or tablets can actually make you feel exhausted faster and your sporting performance worse! (Please see the section on sugar and glucose Chapter 4.) The only exception to this is a professional athlete involved in a marathon or triathlon, where after two hours their body's energy supplies become low and they need to top them up.

If you really want more energy for a sporting event, eat more complex carbohydrates for a couple of days beforehand. This is known as 'carbo-loading'. Get a good night's sleep the night before. Don't eat any closer than two hours before you exercise as your blood supply will be busy digesting the food instead of dedicating itself to your muscles.

Finally, it is worth repeating that exercise really is a miracle activity which will probably do more for you than anything else in this book. **Get moving!**

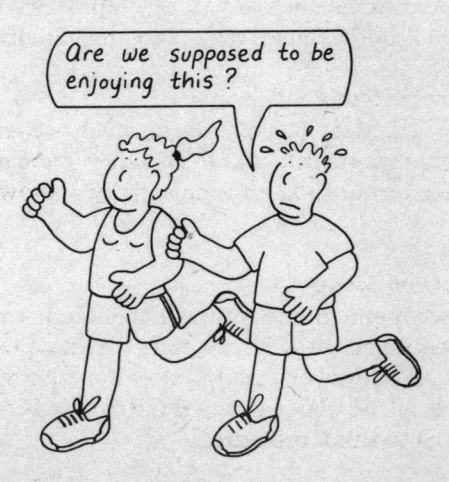

Index

The letter t after page numbers indicates table

abortion 95
abuse 83
acne *see* spots
Acne Support Group 22
aerobic exercise *see* exercise
AIDS 96
alcohol 52, 61, 62, 87–9, 107
Alcoholics Anonymous 85, 90
anaerobic exercise 115
anorexia nervosa 38, 64–5, 67–70, 75
Anti-Bullying Campaign 82
anti-cancer diets 61–2
antibiotics
   and treatment of acne 20
antihistamines 107
appetite 63–4 *see also* eating disorders
ASH 92
attractiveness
   found in girls by boys 40–1

benzoyl peroxide 18–19
birth control *see* contraception
blackheads 10–11, 13, 15, 16
BMI (body mass index) 44–5, 46–7t
boarding schools 81
body clock 103–4

body fat *see* fat, body
body mass index (BMI) 42–43, 44–5t, 47
body shape **36–47**
   being slim 39–41
   and exercise 116
   of models 36–9
   and smoking 90
   waist-to-hip ratio 43, 46t
   see also dieting; weight
boils 12, 21
breakfast
   importance of in diet 57–8
Brook helpline 95
bulimia nervosa 38, 64–5, 70–3, 75
bullying 81–2, 114

caffeine 106–7
calcium 60–1, 62
calisthenics 117, 118
calories 48–9, 50, 51–2, 116
cancer
   anti-cancer diets 61–2
   skin 24–5, 26, 27
carbohydrates 107, 121
   importance in diet 51–2, 54
   source of energy 48–9, 60
Childline 79

chlamydia 96
chocolate
    in diet 12, 54, 106
    effect on spots 12, 14
cholesterol 50
circuit training 118
clothing
    protection from sun 29
    and skin 16
compulsive eating 64, 75
condoms 96, 97, 98
contraception 94, 95 see also
    condoms
contraceptive pill
    and acne 14, 21
cosmetics see make-up
creams, spot, 13, 18–19
cysts 21

dance drugs 92
depression 77, 112
diet 12–13, 57–61
    principles of healthy 62
dieting 38, 50, 66
    disadvantages of 43, 47
diets
    anti-cancer 61–2
    high-protein 59
    low-fat 47, 52–4
    vegetarian 56–7
doctors
    advice on acne 19–20
    advice on family planning
        95–6
drinking see alcohol
drinks, sports 59–60, 121
drugs 92–3, 107

eating see food
eating disorders 38, **63–75**
    causes 65–7
    harm caused by 71–2
    help for 73–5
    see also anorexia nervosa;
        bulimia nervosa
Ecstasy 92
endorphins 105, 111

energy
    and exercise 113
    and sugar 59–60
exam performance, improving
    100–9, 112
    and exercise 105
    importance of sleep 103–4
    and nutrition 106–7
    stress 108–9
exercise **110–121**
    benefits of 110, 112–14
    and exam performance 105
    and good health 47, 52
    muscle strengthening 117–18
    weight loss 52, 115–17
eyes
    protection from sunlight 34

face
    make-up 15, 17
    washing of 13, 17
    see also spots
Family Planning Association 95
fat, body 49–50, 58
    and alcohol 88
    reduction of
        through diet 51–2
        through exercise 115–17
fat, dietary 49
    and cancer 61
    reduction in your diet 52–5
    types of 50–1
figure see body shape
food **48–62**
    and acne 12–13
    basic elements of 48–9
    see also diet; diets; eating
        disorders
food labels 54–55t, 62

gay relationships 83–5, 94, 97
genital warts 96
glue sniffing 93
GP see doctors

hair, greasy
    and spots 15

INDEX

Hepatitis B 97
high-protein diets 59
homosexuals *see* gay relationships

intrauterine device (IUD) 94
isometric exercises 117
isotretinoin tablets 21

lesbian *see* gay relationships
Lifeline 93
lotions
    for control of acne 20
    suntan 27–9
low-fat diet 47, 52–4
LSD (Acid) 92

make-up 15, 17
malignant melanoma 27
masturbation 97–8
menstruation
    protection during 98–9
minerals 49
models
    and body shape 37, 39–40
muscle 115–17
    strengthening of 59, 117–18
music
    effect on studying 107–8
myths
    about diet 57–61
    causes of spots 12–13

NSPCC 83
nutrition
    and exam performance 106–7

obesity 58, 116
oestrogen tablets 21
over-eating 64, 75
ozone layer 25

parents 85
    and diet 57
    and eating disorders 65–6
    and exams 108–9
    and smoking 91–2

periods *see* menstruation
pill, contraceptive
    and acne 14, 21
polyunsaturates 50, 53
pregnancy 94–5
protein 49, 51, 59

Resolve 93
Retin-A 20

salt 62
Samaritans 79
sanitary towels 98–9
saturates 50
sex 90–1, 93–8 *see also* gay relationships
sexually transmitted diseases (STDs) 96–7
skin
    effect of sun on 23–7
    spots *see* spots
skin cancer 24, 26, 27
sleep 103–4
slimness 39–42, 67 *see also* dieting
smoking 89–92
snacks 54, 58
soaps 13, 17
solvent abuse 93
SPF (Sun Protection Factor) 30–1, 32t 33
sport *see* exercise
sports drinks 59–60, 121
spots **9–22**
    causes 10–17
    control of 17–21
    removal of 16–17
    and suntans 17, 29
starches *see* carbohydrates
STD (sexually transmitted diseases) 96–7
stress
    and acne 14
    effect of exercise on 112
    in exams 101, 108–9
studying *see* exam performance, improving

sugar
  in blood 60, 106
  in food and drink 59–60, 67, 121
suicide 78–9
Sun Protection Factor (SPF) 30–33
sunbeds 27, 34
sunburn 26–7, 29
  protection against 30–4
  relief from 35
sunglasses 34
sunscreens 28–30, 30–4
suntan **23–35**
  effect on acne 17, 29
  effect of sun on skin 23–7
  protection 29–34

tampons 98–9
tan *see* suntan
television
  effect on exam study 107–8
  linked to obesity 58
testosterone 10
tetracyclines 20
topical antibiotics 20
toxic shock syndrome (TSS) 99
tretinoin 20

ultraviolet radiation
  protection against 29–34
  UBV and UVA rays 25–6, 27
unhappiness **76–85**

variable resistance machines 118
vegans 56–7
vegetarian diet 56–7
vitamins 49, 59, 107

waist-to-hip ratio (WHR) 43, 46t, 47
washing, face 13, 17
water calisthenics 118
weight **36–47**, 57–8
  dieting *see* dieting
  finding your body mass index 42–3, 44–5t, 47
  losing 47, 51–2, 53–4
weight training 118
WHR (waist-to-hip ratio) 43, 46t, 47
Women's Environmental Network 99
worry
  over exams 108–9
writing
  of problems 80–1

Other *BBC Books* available from
the Going Live! series include:

EMMA FORBES' GOING LIVE! COOKBOOK

MORE LETTERS TO GROWING PAINS
by Phillip Hodson

GROWING PAINS
by Phillip Hodson

GOING LIVE! CAT BOOK
by Grace McHattie

GOING LIVE! PET BOOK
by Nigel Taylor